MAKING  AL

MAKING SENSE OF YOUR SURGICAL ATTACHMENT

Paul Sutton
BMedSci (Hons) BMBS (Hons),
Junior Doctor at Derby City Hospital and President
of SCRUBS in 2005/6

Polly Drew
BMedSci (Hons), 2006/7 President of SCRUBS

Rebecca Lee
BMedSci (Hons), 2006/7 Vice-President of SCRUBS

Michele Chimenti
BMedSci (Hons),
Clinical Co-ordinator on the 2006/7 SCRUBS committee

David Lee
BMedSci (Hons),
Clinical Co-ordinator on the 2006/7 SCRUBS committee

The authors all undertook their medical and surgical training at
the University of Nottingham Medical School. SCRUBS is the
University of Nottingham's Surgical Society

Editorial Advisor: Michael Larvin
FRCS, Professor of Surgery at Nottingham
University and responsible for the Surgeons in Training Education
Programme (STEP) at the Royal College of Surgeons of England

Hodder Arnold

www.hoddereducation.com

First published in Great Britain in 2008 by
Hodder Arnold, an imprint of Hodder Education and a member of the Hachette
Livre UK Group, 338 Euston Road, London NW1 3BH

http://www.hoddereducation.com

Hachette Livre UK's policy is to use papers that are natural, renewable and
recyclable products and made from wood grown in sustainable forests. The logging
and manufacturing processes are expected to conform to the environmental
regulations of the country of origin.

Whilst the advice and information in this book are believed to be true and accurate
at the date of going to press, neither the author[s] nor the publisher can accept any
legal responsibility or liability for any errors or omissions that may be made. In
particular, (but without limiting the generality of the preceding disclaimer) every
effort has been made to check drug dosages; however it is still possible that errors
have been missed. Furthermore, dosage schedules are constantly being revised and
new side-effects recognized. For these reasons the reader is strongly urged to
consult the drug companies' printed instructions before administering any of the
drugs recommended in this book.

British Library Cataloguing in Publication Data
A catalogue record for this book is available from the British Library

Library of Congress Cataloging-in-Publication Data
A catalog record for this book is available from the Library of Congress

ISBN   978-0-340-94588-9

1 2 3 4 5 6 7 8 9 10

Commissioning Editor:	Sara Purdy
Project Editor:	Jane Tod
Production Controller:	Lindsay Smith
Cover Design:	Laura de Grasse
Indexer:	Indexing Specialists (UK) Ltd

Typeset in 10.5/13 RotisSerif by Charon Tec Ltd (A MacMillan Company)
www.chartontec.com
Printed and bound in Spain

What do you think about this book? Or any other Hodder Arnold title?
Please visit our website: www.hoddereducation.com

For my mum, dad, sister and Lucy.
PS

To Robina and Nigel, without you I wouldn't be where
I am today. Thank you for your continued love, support and
guidance.
PD

Per la famiglia Chimenti e Anna.
MC

Thanks to mum, dad and Andy.
RL, DL

CONTENTS

Foreword   ix
Introduction from the Editor   xi
Acknowledgements   xiii
List of abbreviations   xv

1   Perioperative care   1
2   Anaesthesia and the anaesthetic room   20
3   The operating theatre   38
4   Scrubbing up   51
5   Surgical instruments   61
6   The art of suturing and assisting   72
7   Electrosurgery   86
8   Minimal access surgery   102
9   Health, safety and surgeons   115
10 You as a trainee   124

Index   143

FOREWORD

It is a pleasure and a privilege to have been asked to write the foreword for this book. The first visit to the operating theatre is a daunting experience for a medical student. Pressure to get cases through the operating theatre in the allocated time often means that the student is ignored or worse still castigated for getting in the way of theatre staff or impinging on sterile equipment. As the editor states in his introduction, there are a lot of 'rules' in surgery which nobody will ever teach you yet everybody will expect you to know.

This book describes theatre etiquette and introduces the student to the layout of theatres, instruments, scrubbing up, assisting, suturing and the principles and practice of laparoscopic surgery. The authors all undertook, or are undertaking, their training at the University of Nottingham School of Medicine. At the time of writing, the senior author and editor was a pre-registration house office (F1), and the authors final year medical students. All the authors are, or have been, associated with SCRUBS, the University of Nottingham Student Surgical Society, one of many student surgical societies developing around the country, supported by the Medical Student Liaison Committee of the Royal College of Surgeons of England. The idea for the book was conceived in 2006 following discussions with colleagues, nurse educators and other medical students about how daunting the operating theatre can be to a medical student. The book that has developed from the embryonic ideas is a gem. It clearly and concisely describes all that the medical student needs to know about the operating theatre in an easy to read manner. This book is an outstanding example of what a group of medical students can achieve when taking control of the ownership of their own learning and disseminating it to their colleagues. Not only will this small volume be invaluable for medical students, but also for basic surgical trainees as a revision book. The authors, who are at an embryonic stage in their career, are to be congratulated. With trainees like these, I think the future of surgery in this country will be safe in their hands. They should be proud of their achievement. I only wish there had been such a book when I was a medical student.

Andrew T Raftery
Chairman
Medical Student Liaison Group
Royal College of Surgeons of England
2008

INTRODUCTION FROM THE EDITOR

Experiences as a medical student vary widely between students, year groups and medical schools. There are lots of reasons for this, but I believe the biggest reason is a student's lack of knowledge regarding how to study throughout their clinical years, and in particular how to make the most of their clinical attachments.

Surgical attachments make up roughly half of a medical school's general curriculum. Many good students find surgery highly daunting, partly due to its rapid pace, but also the added mystique of the operating theatre. People constantly shouting at you to do this or not to do that, not knowing what to touch or not touch, where to stand, when to speak . . . a few bad experiences are enough to put students off for life (or at least the rest of their attachment!).

There are lots of 'rules' in surgery which for some reason no-one will ever teach you, yet everyone expects you to know. This can prevent students from learning effectively during their surgical attachments, and therefore lead to poor performance in subsequent assessments.

You will find this book a compelling guide to help you navigate through your surgical attachments, including the mysteries of 'theatre'. It will also ensure that you enjoy your surgical attachments and obtain the best possible learning from them – whether you are thinking of pursuing a surgical career or not. Importantly, if you do decide on a career in surgery, it will help you on your way to success.

Paul Sutton
2008

ACKNOWLEDGEMENTS

The authors would like to formally acknowledge the following for their assistance in the production of this book:

Professor Mike Larvin

Dr Gareth Moncaster

Mr Simon Baker

Dr Richard Wain

Mr Andrew Raftery

Dr Lucy Smith

Mr David Foreman

Miss Alex Hart

LIST OF ABBREVIATIONS

AC	alternating current
ASA	American Society of Anesthesiologists
CCT	Certificate of Completion of Training
CUSA	Cavitron Ultrasonic Surgical Aspirator
DC	direct current
DVT/PE	deep vein thrombosis/pulmonary embolism
ECG	electrocardiogram
ED	emergency department
ERCP	endoscopic retrograde cholangio-pancreatography
ETT	endotracheal tube
FBC	full blood count
GCS	Glasgow Coma Score
HDU	high-dependency unit
HEPA	high-efficiency particulate air
Hz	hertz
INR	international normalized ratio
IRMER	Ionising Radiation (Medical Exposure) Regulations
ITU	intensive therapy unit
IV	intravenous
IVRA	intravenous regional anaesthesia
LLETZ	large loop excision of transformation zone
LMA	laryngeal mask airway
MEWS	modified early warning score
MMC	Modernising Medical Careers
MRSA	methicillin-resistant *Staphylococcus aureus*

MTAS	Medical Training Application Service
MUA	manipulation under anaesthesia
NICE	National Institute for Health and Clinical Excellence
NOTES	natural orifice transluminal endoscopic surgery
NSAID	non-steroidal anti-inflammatory drug
ODPs	operating department practitioner
OGD	oesophagogastroduodenoscopy
PDS	polydioxanone
PRHO	pre-registration house officer
RSI	rapid sequence induction
SHO	senior house officer
SpR	specialist registrar
ST	specialty training
StR	specialist trainee
TLD	thermoluminescent dosimeter
VATS	video-assisted thoracoscopic surgery

1

PERIOPERATIVE CARE

The perioperative period refers to the time surrounding a patient's surgical procedure – from hospitalization to discharge. It can be divided into three distinct phases: preoperative, intraoperative and postoperative.

REFERRAL AND PREOPERATIVE ASSESSMENT

Referral for surgical procedures may come from many sources, most usually general practitioners, physicians, the emergency department or from other hospitals. Any patient who requires a surgical procedure will need to undergo a preoperative assessment. For elective (planned) procedures, this assessment aims to ensure that the patient's health is optimized before surgery. Emergency patients also require preoperative assessment, but on a more rapid time-scale (Box 1.1).

The location and timing of preoperative assessment is variable and can occur at any time between the patient giving their consent to a surgical procedure and the date of the agreed operation. The methods used to carry out a preoperative assessment vary from hospital to hospital. Within the UK this may involve any combination of the following:

- Anaesthetic outpatient clinic
- Surgical outpatient clinic
- Specialized preoperative assessment clinic

Box 1.1 NCEPOD scoring

The National Confidential Enquiry into Patient Outcome and
Death (NCEPOD) suggested that a classification system to
identify the urgency of a patient's intervention be used, and that
every acute hospital have a designated emergency theatre.

1	Immediate	Life, limb, or organ threatening (resuscitation simultaneous with surgical treatment)
2A	Within 6 hours	Emergency surgery once patient stabilized
2B	Within 24 hours	Urgent surgery once patient stabilized
3	Expedited	Stable patient requiring early intervention for a condition which is not an immediate risk to life, limb, or organ
4	Elective	Planned or booked surgery

- Inpatient assessment
- Medical questionnaire.

The assessment may be carried out by any trained medical
professional, commonly a junior member of the surgical team,
an anaesthetist or trained nurse.

The format for the assessment follows the structure of *history,
examination, investigations* and *consent.*

Key point

Last minute assessments carried out on the patient in the
anaesthetic room should be avoided if at all possible.
Emergency patients must be fully resuscitated before arrival.

HISTORY

The history should cover the following points:

- Name/age/occupation
- Past medical history

- Drug history and allergies
- Anaesthetic and surgical history
- Family history
- Social history
- Dental work.

Past medical history

Any physiological system within the body can affect, and be affected by, anaesthesia (Box 1.2). It is therefore important to take a detailed past medical history to assess any risk factors that may be present. The cardiovascular and respiratory systems are particularly important within the context of preoperative assessment and should be the focus of the history. The following conditions are clearly associated with increased anaesthetic risk and should be specifically asked about.

Cardiovascular system

- Ischaemic heart disease: higher risk of intraoperative or postoperative death
- Heart failure: increased risk of cardiac morbidity and mortality

---

Box 1.2   American Society of Anesthesiologists (ASA) physical status classification system

The ASA scoring system categorizes patients into five subgroups by preoperative physical fitness:

I   A completely healthy patient
II   A patient with mild systemic disease
III A patient with severe systemic disease that is not incapacitating
IV   A patient with incapacitating disease that is a constant threat to life
V   A moribund patient who is not expected to live 24 hours with or without surgery.

The suffix 'E' is used to indicate an emergency case.

- Hypertension: risk of myocardial and cerebral ischaemia
- Arrhythmias
- Peripheral vascular disease.

Key symptoms and signs to consider are: chest pain, palpitations, orthopnoea, breathlessness (particularly at night), exercise tolerance and ankle swelling.

> ### Key point
>
> Unless critical, surgery should not be performed on a patient who has suffered a myocardial infarction within the last six months, due to the risk of re-infarction.

Respiratory system

- Chronic obstructive airways disease
- Emphysema
- Asthma
- Respiratory infection
- Restrictive lung disease.

Any patient with a pre-existing lung condition is more susceptible to developing a respiratory tract infection postoperatively.

Key symptoms and signs to consider are: cough, sputum, wheeze, shortness of breath and cyanosis.

Other systems

Neurological system

- Stroke: increased risk of further stroke.

Endocrine system

- Diabetes: increased incidence of cardiovascular and renal complications
- Adrenal insufficiency: additional steroid cover may be required.

Alimentary system

- Hiatal hernia: increased risk of regurgitation and aspiration
- Liver cirrhosis: interference with drug metabolism and impaired blood clotting.

Genitourinary system

- Renal failure: altered drug excretion may restrict the use of certain anaesthetic agents
- Pregnancy: anaesthetic agents used in early pregnancy may be teratogenic.

Haematological system

- Clotting disorders: increased or uncontrollable blood loss
- Sickle cell disease: incorrect anaesthetic techniques may result in hypoxia and precipitate a sickle cell crisis, as may the use of a surgical tourniquet.

Musculoskeletal system

- Rheumatoid arthritis: restriction of neck and jaw movements may hinder airway management, and atlanto-axial instability requires caution.

Nutrition

- Obesity: increases risk of surgical and airway management, respiratory tract infection, deep vein thrombosis/pulmonary embolism (DVT/PE), delayed wound healing
- Cachexia/malnutrition: increases surgical risk and hinders healing and recovery
- Vitamin or trace element deficiency: delays healing
- Anaemia: reduces tolerance to effects of operative blood loss, and delays healing.

Drug history

All current drugs and medications should be recorded, detailing the dose, route of administration and frequency. Allergies to drugs, latex, elastoplast, iodine and dressings should be enquired about, and documented. Ask specifically about the oral contraceptive pill, which can increase the risk of DVT and PE, as many patients will forget this or think that it is unimportant.

Drugs that pose a particular risk to anaesthesia and surgery include the following:

● Steroids: associated with adrenocorticoid suppression
● Antibiotics: can prolong the action of muscle relaxants used
● Monoamine oxidase inhibitors: interaction with opiates may cause severe tachycardia and hypertension
● Warfarin: risk of increased blood loss during surgery.

Anaesthetic and surgical history

Any previous history of operations (dental or surgical) and anaesthetics should be well documented. The following should be considered:

● What surgery was performed and why?
● Were there any difficulties in obtaining an airway?
● Which anaesthetic agents and techniques were used and were they well tolerated?
● Did the patient exhibit any signs of allergic reaction to drugs used?
● Did the patient experience any postoperative complications?
● Is there any history of scoline apnoea (persistent neuromuscular blockade following suxamethonium)?

Postoperative complications (for example nausea, vomiting, sore throat) and difficulty performing procedures, such as intubation, are important to establish as they may influence subsequent management of the patient's anaesthesia.

Family history

Certain hereditary conditions can influence the anaesthetic management of a patient. An accurate family history is particularly important in patients who are undergoing their first surgical procedure. Conditions to be aware of and to seek in the family history during a preoperative assessment include:

● Sickle cell disease
● Malignant hyperpyrexia

- Porphyrias
- Dystrophia myotonica
- Haemoglobinopathies
- Cholinesterase abnormalities.

Social history

The most important features of the social history are smoking, alcohol and illicit drug use. Smoking should be recorded in 'pack years'. One pack year is equivalent to one pack of 20 cigarettes a day for one year. Two pack years is equivalent to 20 cigarettes a day for two years, 40 cigarettes a day for one year, or any other combination.

Alcohol consumption should be recorded in units per week (1 unit is half a pint of standard strength beer, a small glass of wine or one measure of spirit).

Recreational drug use should also be enquired about, specifically the substance used, frequency of its use and route of administration. You may have to reassure patients that this information is confidential but vital for their safe care, as well as that of the staff caring for them.

Smoking

Cigarette smoke contains carbon monoxide, which combines with haemoglobin in the blood to form carboxyhaemoglobin. This form of haemoglobin has reduced oxygen-carrying capacity and its presence increases the likelihood of hypoxia. Additionally, nicotine activates the sympathetic nervous system, resulting in tachycardia, hypertension and constriction of the coronary arteries.

Patients should be encouraged to stop smoking, ideally several weeks prior to their surgical procedure, and help should be offered to them in order to achieve this.

Alcohol

An alcohol intake in excess of approximately 50 units a week is associated with liver enzyme induction, which may alter the action of anaesthetic drugs.

Recreational drug use

Withdrawal and difficulties with venous access are important considerations for patients who are known drug users.

Dental work

During anaesthetic induction a patient will require maintenance of their airway. Caps, false teeth and poor dental work can increase the difficulty in securing a patient's airway and should be notified to the anaesthetist prior to induction.

EXAMINATION

The examination should be directed by the history and should focus on the cardiovascular and respiratory systems. Additional systems are examined if problems relevant to anaesthesia have been identified during history taking. A neurological examination, for example, would be appropriate in a patient who has had a stroke.

To complete the examination all patients must undergo a full assessment of their airway.

Airway assessment

The patient's airway should be assessed to determine the ease or otherwise of endotracheal intubation. During endotracheal intubation a tube is introduced, usually through the oropharynx and into the trachea, to protect the patient's airway while they are unconscious. The procedure requires the patient's neck to be extended back and their mouth opened so that the tube can be guided into the trachea.

The following should be considered as part of the airway assessment:

● Degree of mouth opening
● Size and position of the mandible
● Size of the tongue

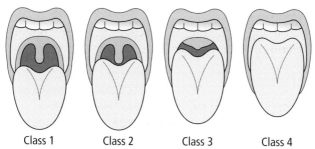

Figure 1.1 The Mallampati classification used to predict difficult intubation. It is based on the structures visualized when the mouth is opened wide and tongue protruding

● Location and quality of the teeth, presence of false teeth, caps and crowns
● Any limitations of cervical spine movement (flexion/ extension).

Measurements are commonly made by anaesthetists during the airway assessment as a predictor of difficult intubation. Mallampati grading uses a visual system to assess the vertical distance between the tongue and soft palate (Figure 1.1). There are four grades or classes: 1–4. Thyromental distance is the measurement between the thyroid cartilage and the bony prominence of the mentum (chin) taken with the neck in full extension.

A thyromental distance of less than 7 cm and a Mallampati score of greater than 3 predicts difficult intubation.

Key point

An airway assessment should be performed for every patient, even if intubation is not planned as part of their anaesthetic.

INVESTIGATIONS

The National Institute for Health and Clinical Excellence (NICE) in the UK has published recommendations to try and

Table 1.1 Suggested baseline investigations prior to surgery

Age	Minor procedure	Major procedure
16–40	None	FBC, renal function tests, blood glucose, (clotting)
41–60	ECG	FBC, renal function tests, blood glucose, ECG, (clotting)
61–80	ECG	FBC, renal function tests, blood glucose, ECG, chest X-ray, (clotting)
>80	ECG, FBC, renal function tests	FBC, renal function tests, blood glucose, ECG, chest X-ray, clotting

FBC, full blood count; ECG, electrocardiogram.

 standardize preoperative investigations (www.nice.org.uk/cg3). Your own hospital, however, may have its own variants. Investigations should be based on the history and examination, and used only when there is a significant chance of detecting an abnormality that may influence surgery and/or anaesthesia.

In patients with no concurrent medical conditions, the baseline investigations required will depend on the patient's age and the type of surgery to be performed (Table 1.1).

It is not common practice to perform further investigations unless specifically indicated. For example, if a murmur is detected, an echocardiogram is indicated and should be arranged. If the patient has a history of fibrotic lung disease, lung function testing should be performed.

CONSENT

The responsibility for obtaining consent rests with the surgeon responsible for the operative procedure. For consent to be valid (legally binding) the patient must make an informed decision based upon up-to-date and accurate information relating to the risks, benefits and possible complications of the proposed procedure. The patient must also be competent to understand and retain this information.

The process of gaining consent is usually performed in the following manner:

- Establish the patient's current level of understanding
- Explain the condition and treatment options
- Explain the proposed intervention
- Explain the benefits, risks, complications and alternatives to the proposed intervention
- Explain the natural history without intervention
- Answer any questions
- Evaluate their capacity
- Summarize
- Complete the consent form, which is then signed by both parties.

> ### Key point
>
> Taking consent is a serious responsibility, and trainees should never undertake to do this unless they have been adequately trained to do so.

PREPARATION FOR THEATRE

After the preoperative assessment the patient goes home, and will not normally return until the day of their procedure.

Should any further preparation be required prior to the procedure, the patient may need to be admitted to hospital earlier. For example, a patient established on warfarin therapy may need to be transferred to a heparin infusion. Heparin has a short half-life and is more easily reversed than warfarin if ongoing anticoagulation is required (e.g. in a patient with a metallic heart valve). It is usually stopped a few hours preoperatively, and recommenced shortly afterwards. On cessation of warfarin, the INR (international normalized ratio) should be less than 1.5 for safe surgery.

A second example would be insulin-dependent diabetic patients. They are frequently brought in either the day before surgery or early on the day of surgery to be established on a continuous intravenous insulin infusion, referred to as a sliding scale, in order to optimize glycaemic control.

Some preparation may be conducted at home. The most common example of this is bowel preparation to 'cleanse' the bowel prior to surgery. This is an attempt to minimize the consequences of leakage from a colonic anastomosis (surgical join). A recent Cochrane Systematic Review (www. thecochranelibrary.com) questioned the efficacy of 'bowel prep', but you will find it still commonly employed in UK hospitals.

On the day of surgery

Patients must be starved of solids and coloured fluids (for example milk, fizzy and hot drinks) for 6 hours, and clear fluids for 2 hours prior to surgery in order to minimize the risk of aspiration. They must also change into a hospital gown and remove all jewellery, metallic and personal items. Nail varnish should also be removed as this may interfere with pulse oximetry readings.

A review of the patient's medication should take place. Certain drugs, such as aspirin and non-steroidal anti-inflammatory drugs (NSAIDs) need to be temporarily stopped as they may increase bleeding.

A brief respiratory examination needs to be performed to exclude major acute respiratory tract infection, as this may be a contraindication to general anaesthesia.

Finally, the patient should be given the opportunity to ask any remaining questions, and his or her understanding of the procedure should be double checked to ensure that consent remains valid. The nursing staff on the ward will ensure that the patient is sent to theatre with the notes, investigation results, drug card and consent form.

> ## Key point
>
> The site of the operation should be marked by the operating surgeon whilst the patient is conscious. It should be checked against the notes, consent form, theatre list and with the patient directly.

Preoperative removal of hair at the operative site is no longer carried out routinely, but may sometimes be necessary, for example in neurosurgical procedures. A Cochrane Systematic Review (www.thecochranelibrary.com) found little difference between shaving, clipping and chemical depilation, but shaving was found to be best carried out in the operating theatre rather than preoperatively.

Some hospitals use a procedure-specific wrist band, on which the type and side of operation are written and signed by patient and surgeon. Whether this system is in place or not, the patient must be identified and their details checked by the operating surgeon prior to anaesthesia. It is reassuring for a patient to be greeted personally by their surgeon.

After moving into theatre it is a good idea to have a final 'STOP' moment, where all activity ceases so that the team can carry out one last check that the correct procedure is being performed on the correct patient.

Preoperative medications

Drugs administered prior to induction of anaesthesia are less commonly used nowadays, as they are no longer part of the anaesthetic drug regimen. Drugs most commonly used include the following:

● Anxiolytics, such as lorazepam, temazepam and midazolam. These act to reduce anxiety.
● Analgesics, such as morphine and pethidine. Opioid analgesia is used for patients who are in pain preoperatively, especially emergency patients.

- Anticholinergics, such as atropine and glycopyrrolate. These act to reduce salivation. They also have a cardiac vagolytic effect which may lead to tachycardia.
- Antacids, such as ranitidine and omeprazole. If a patient has not undergone adequate preoperative fasting or is at increased risk of aspiration due to obesity or hiatal hernia, these drugs may help to reduce the risk of aspiration.
- Antiemetics, such as cyclizine and metoclopramide. Administration of an opioid analgesic is commonly associated with nausea and vomiting. Prescription of an antiemetic may help to prevent post-op nausea and vomiting.
- Antibiotic prophylaxis, such as a cephalosporin and metronidazole for gastrointestinal tract surgery. Each hospital has its own specific protocol.

In addition the patient should receive all his or her usual medication unless they have been altered for the purpose of surgery, for example the conversion of oral steroids to intravenous hydrocortisone.

INDUCTION OF ANAESTHESIA AND THE INTRAOPERATIVE PERIOD

The final stage in preparation for surgery is the induction of anaesthesia. Following this the anaesthesia needs to be maintained, and the patient closely monitored while the procedure is performed. This is known as the intraoperative period, and is discussed in detail in Chapter 2.

THE POSTOPERATIVE PERIOD

Patients are monitored very closely during the intraoperative period, however most complications of anaesthesia and surgery occur postoperatively. For this reason it is vital that the patient receives close attention and care during the recovery period.

The recovery period

The recovery period describes the period of time after the patient leaves the direct supervision of the anaesthetist and is transferred from theatre, usually to a recovery unit situated within the theatre area. The role of the anaesthetist does not cease, however, as the patient remains the anaesthetist's responsibility until he or she is discharged from the recovery area back to the ward.

The recovery ward is a specialized area located close to theatres, equipped with trained staff and equipment to deal with any complication that may be encountered postoperatively. All recovery areas should be equipped with the following:

- Oxygen supply
- Suction
- ECG monitoring
- Pulse oximetry
- Blood pressure monitoring
- Equipment for the management of an obstructed airway
- Ventilation equipment
- Resuscitation equipment (e.g. defibrillator)
- Drugs for post-op pain relief, anaesthesia and resuscitation
- An alarm system to summon anaesthetic assistance.

Key point

A patient unable to maintain his or her airway should never be left unsupervised.

Critical care areas

A patient usually spends a minimum of 30 minutes in recovery, but the length of admission varies from patient to patient. For discharge to occur the following criteria must be fulfilled:

1. The patient is fully conscious (ideally GCS 15)
2. The patient is able to maintain their own airway

3. Respiratory rate and oxygenation are normal
4. Cardiovascular system is satisfactory and stable
5. Bleeding is absent or controlled
6. Pain management and nausea are controlled
7. The patient is warm.

Once the patient has met the minimum discharge criteria they may be transferred out of recovery.

Transfer locations include surgical wards, the intensive therapy unit (ITU), or high-dependency unit (HDU). The HDU is a compromise between ITU and the ward areas, which can provide a higher level of care and is sometimes known as a 'Step Down' unit. A patient's destination will depend upon the procedure performed, preoperative morbidity, the presence or increased risk of any complications and their progress so far in recovery.

Postoperative care

Postoperative care of the patient involves the frequent checking of vital signs such as pulse rate, blood pressure, urine output, respiratory rate, oxygen saturations and conscious level. Each hospital will have a protocol for routine postoperative observations, typically quarter-hourly for 1 hour, half-hourly for 2 hours, and perhaps hourly for 6–12 hours thereafter, depending on the procedure. Should problems arise the patient may be transferred to a modified early warning score (MEWS) chart, and if sufficient physiological abnormalities lead to a high MEWS rating, an ITU opinion will be triggered automatically.

In addition to these, specific checks relevant to the procedure performed should be undertaken, such as the level of epidural block, output from drains, the site of the wound and/or stoma, and the presence of distal pulses in vascular and orthopaedic surgery. These checks are usually performed by a designated nurse.

The surgical team will perform daily ward rounds to monitor the patient's progress and assess other aspects such as wound healing and drain output, returning at the nurses' request to review patients with possible complications.

Physiotherapists will see any patient with chest complications, or who require special exercises, for example orthopaedic patients. Patients on ITU/HDU will also be seen frequently by an intensivist (usually an anaesthetic consultant).

An outreach nurse from ITU will usually continue to visit recently discharged patients to check whether readmission to ITU is required.

Early mobilization and discharge has been shown to improve outcomes and, in particular, may help reduce cross-infection risk. Discharge planning usually commences at the preadmission assessment, taking into account domestic circumstances and socio-economic factors.

Wound drains may have been placed to prevent the intra-abdominal accumulation of serum or lymph, or to warn and protect against the leakage of bile, gastric, or pancreatic juice. Their removal is generally decided upon by the operating surgeon, and is usually performed when they 'dry' or reduce below a certain level, such as 30 mL/day. Urinary catheters are usually removed when patients are ambulant or when close monitoring is no longer required.

Day case surgery is becoming more popular and is associated with reduced complication risks, but requires that adequate oral pain relief is provided, a responsible carer is present with the patient for at least 24 hours, and there must be telephone access to the hospital. Overnight stay surgery has become the norm for non-major procedures, with discharge home the following day.

Follow-up

Prior to discharge from hospital, follow-up appointments with the patient's surgical team may be required to monitor progress. The level of monitoring and frequency of follow-up appointments will vary depending on the type of surgical procedure performed. For example, a patient who has undergone a colectomy will require more intensive follow-up than a patient who has undergone a simple hernia repair.

Sutures or staples requiring removal are less commonly employed these days, but if they are used, arrangements must be made for removal by a district or practice nurse. Wounds are often closed using subcuticular techniques (see Chapter 6) or glued so as not to require stitch removal. Wounds should be inspected prior to discharge to ensure that bleeding has ceased and that there are no early signs of wound infection (erythema or discharge of pus).

Finally, discharge medication must be prescribed and a discharge letter written for the patient's GP, who is nowadays most likely to be the doctor who deals with any postoperative complications.

Postoperative complications

Only a minority of patients develop complications after their surgery. Common problems include:

- Postoperative nausea and vomiting
- Pain
- Sore throat from airway management
- Hypoxaemia
- Hyper/hypotension
- Poor urine output
- Bleeding
- Infection
- Wound complications
- Deep complications at the site of surgery.

Complications from surgery are classically divided into anaesthetic or surgical, and subclassified as immediate, short term and long term. They vary considerably between procedures.

Summary

● Thorough preoperative assessment is vital to ensure a positive outcome.

● Obtaining valid consent is an important skill.

● Investigations are not routine but should be directed towards the patient.

● The patient should be thoroughly prepared for theatre.

● The recovery period is an important part of the patient's journey.

● Close postoperative monitoring is essential in order to check on progress.

2

ANAESTHESIA AND THE ANAESTHETIC ROOM

In this chapter we discuss anaesthesia and the techniques and drugs involved. We will also describe the anaesthetic room and the equipment and resources that you will encounter in this setting.

INTRODUCTION

Anaesthesia is the loss of feeling in all or part of the body. It can be caused by trauma or disease, but in the context of surgery it refers to the technique of reducing bodily sensation to pain to allow surgical procedures to be carried out. The effect of anaesthesia can be achieved across the whole body using a general anaesthetic, or restricted to a localized region by use of a regional anaesthetic technique. The decision to use a general, regional or local technique will depend upon various factors, including the type and site of the operation, the patient's physical health and the experience and preference of the anaesthetist and surgeon.

Anaesthesia is commonly referred to in terms of stages:

- Stage 1 Analgesia: This stage ends with loss of consciousness.

- Stage 2 Excitation: Breath holding, coughing and pupillary dilation may be observed.
- Stage 3 Surgical anaesthesia: Reduced respiratory and muscular activity. This stage concludes with loss of diaphragmatic activity.
- Stage 4 Respiratory and cardiac failure: Vital brainstem reflexes are impaired by high concentrations of anaesthetic agents. Pupils become fixed and dilated.

Key point

Stage 4 of anaesthesia represents an anaesthetic emergency – patients should not reach this stage!

ANAESTHETIC DRUGS

Anaesthetic agents are most commonly delivered either by inhalation or by the intravenous route, although virtually any route of administration can be used:

- Inhalation: induction anaesthetics
- Intravenous: muscle relaxants
- Intramuscular: NSAIDs
- Subcutaneous: opioids
- Intrathecal: opioids
- Rectal: benzodiazepines, NSAIDs
- Topical: EMLA (eutectic mixture of local anaesthetic).

There are several properties that are desirable for anaesthetic drugs, regardless of the route of administration:

- Quick onset of action
- Rapid elimination from the body
- Minimal side-effects
- Wide margin of safety.

A knowledge of some of the more common anaesthetic drugs and the underlying physiology and pharmacology is expected of all trainees, and also of students on their anaesthetic attachments (Table 2.1).

Inhalation anaesthetics

These types of drugs are inhaled into the patient's lungs as a gaseous agent. Once in the lungs they disperse into the alveoli and diffuse into arterial blood to reach the brain. The concentration or partial pressure of the drug within the alveoli is said to equate to that in the cerebral circulation. Changes in alveoli partial pressures therefore will reflect changes in the partial pressure of the drug being delivered to the brain.

The MAC number, commonly associated with inhaled anaesthetic drugs, refers to the minimum alveolar concentration required to prevent response to a surgical stimulus in 50 per cent of patients.

> ### Key point
>
> The MAC figures for anaesthetic agents refer to 50 per cent of patients, therefore many will need higher concentrations than this.

Intravenous anaesthetics

Intravenous (IV) anaesthetics are administered directly into the patient's bloodstream via their venous system. These drugs are commonly administered by syringe through a cannula sited in the dorsum of the patient's hand, and are often referred to as parenteral drugs (i.e. not involving the gastrointestinal tract).

Commonly used IV anaesthetic drugs include:

● Narcotics
● Muscle relaxants
● Reversal agents.

Narcotics

Narcotics (opioids) are used to control perioperative pain and anxiety. Their effects include analgesia, depression of

Table 2.1 Commonly used anaesthetic drugs

Drug class and name	Anaesthetic use	Mode of action
Ethers (isoflurane, sevoflurane)	Inhalation induction	Unknown
Halogenated hydrocarbon (halothane)	Inhalation induction	Unknown
Gaseous molecules (nitrous oxide, Entonox)	Inhalation analgesic and weak induction agent	Unknown
Imidazoles (etomidate)	IV Induction: loss of consciousness	Suppression of neuronal activity
Arylcyclohexylamines (ketamine)	IV Induction: associated with a feeling of dissociation	Unknown
Alkylphenols (propofol)	IV Induction and maintenance of anaesthesia	Suppression of neuronal activity
Benzodiazepines (lorazepam, midazolam, diazepam)	Induction: amnesic agent and minor tranquilizer	Potentiation of GABA (inhibitory neurotransmitter)
Amine ester (suxamethonium)	Muscle relaxant	Depolarizing muscle relaxant
Benzylisoquinolinium (atracurium)	Muscle relaxant	Non-depolarizing muscle relaxant
Aminosteroids (vecuronium, rocuronium)	Muscle relaxant	Non-depolarizing muscle relaxant
Anticholinesterase (neostigmine)	Reversal agent	Antagonist to non-depolarizing relaxant
Antimuscarinics (atropine, glycopyrrolate)	Reversal agent	Antimuscarinic
Sympathomimetic amine (ephedrine, amphetamine)	Management of hypotension	Adrenergic effects
Opioids (morphine, fentanyl, codeine)	Analgesia	Agonistic effect at opioid receptors
NSAIDs (aspirin, ibuprofen, diclofenac)	Analgesia	Inhibition of cyclo-oxygenase pathway
Paracetamol	Analgesia	Unknown
Lidocaine/bupivocaine	Local anaesthesia	Sodium channel blocker

respiratory effect and reduction of sensation to surgical stimuli. In large doses they are also able to induce sleep or stupor.

Narcotics have a highly specific receptor-mediating effect. The receptors affected are known as the opioid receptors: μ (mu), κ (kappa) and σ (sigma). The balance between exogenous agonists (for example morphine), endogenous agonists (for example endorphins) and antagonists (such as naloxone) determines pharmacological effect.

Muscle relaxants
Muscle relaxants, as the name suggests, inhibit muscular contraction. There are two types of muscle relaxants that are commonly used within anaesthesia: non-depolarizing and depolarizing blockers. Both types of agent act at the neuromuscular junction.

Non-depolarizing drugs inhibit the action of acetylcholine (the neurotransmitter responsible for muscular contraction) at the motor endplate.

Depolarizing agents bind to acetylcholine receptors at the motor endplate and cause depolarization for as long as they are bound there. This prevents repolarization and subsequent stimulation of the receptor, thereby preventing muscle contraction.

> ## Key point
>
> There are two types of muscle relaxant: non-depolarizing and depolarizing.

Reversal agents
These drugs are used to reverse the effects of muscle relaxants so that the function of respiratory muscles is restored, allowing a return of spontaneous ventilation.

Anticholinergic drugs increase the concentration of acetylcholine by inhibiting the enzyme responsible for its metabolism, acetylcholinesterase. The increase in acetylcholine, however, may cause hypotension and bradycardia. For this reason an antimuscarinic agent is used in conjunction with the anticholinergic, to combat the possible haemodynamic effects.

Intramuscular/subcutaneous anaesthetics

Intramuscular administration of a drug involves the injection of a substance directly into a muscle by use of a needle and syringe. It is useful for drugs which are only required in small amounts, as larger volumes tend to be painful. Commonly used muscles include deltoid, vastus lateralis and the gluteal muscles. When injecting into the gluteal site, care must be taken to ensure that the sciatic nerve is avoided. This is done by siting the injection in the upper outer quadrant of the buttock.

Subcutaneous injections are administered into the fat layer immediately under the skin, usually in the arm, abdomen or upper leg. The substance then diffuses into local blood capillaries and enters the bloodstream. Local anaesthetic agents, for example lidocaine (lignocaine), are administered by this route.

Key point

Always use the upper outer quadrant when injecting intramuscularly into the gluteal region in order to avoid the sciatic nerve.

ANAESTHETIC TECHNIQUES

Techniques used to achieve anaesthesia will vary according to the demands of the procedure.

General anaesthesia

A general anaesthetic is essentially a drug-induced coma, which results in amnesia, analgesia and muscle relaxation (commonly referred to as the triad of anaesthesia). The process of administering a general anaesthetic is described in detail later in this chapter.

Regional anaesthesia

Regional anaesthesia differs from local anaesthesia in that it blocks specific nerves or groups of nerves, thus covering larger areas than simple local infiltration is able to. Regional techniques may be used:

- as the sole anaesthetic technique for surgery,
- for supplementary analgesia,
- for postoperative pain relief, or
- in the management of chronic pain.

Regional anaesthesia can be classed according to the site at which the anaesthetic agents are administered:

- Intravenous regional anaesthesia (IVRA)
- Central nerve blocks
- Peripheral blocks
- Local anaesthetics.

Intravenous regional anaesthesia

Intravenous regional anaesthesia (IVRA) is the intravenous administration of a local anaesthetic agent into a limb (commonly the upper limb) that has been isolated from the general circulation by use of a double tourniquet in order to prevent systemic toxicity. It is also known as a Bier's block, as he first described this in 1908.

IVRA is used for short procedures on the upper or lower limb (below the elbow and knee) with little postoperative pain (e.g. carpal tunnel decompression).

A cannula is inserted into the dorsum of the hand and the limb is drained by elevation. A tourniquet is placed over a padded area of the limb and a carefully calculated dose of local anaesthetic is injected via the cannula into the limb. Anaesthesia is achieved within 10 minutes and the tourniquet is removed after the procedure. Premature release of tourniquets may deliver a toxic dose of the anaesthetic agent into the general circulation. Prolonged application of the tourniquet may lead to irreversible ischaemia. Tourniquet application times are written on the theatre 'board' so that all staff can see and monitor them.

Central nerve blocks

Central nerve blockade describes the administration of local anaesthetic into the extradural (epidural anaesthesia) or subarachnoid (spinal anaesthesia) spaces. It is used as an alternative to general anaesthesia for procedures below the umbilicus.

The patient is positioned sitting up or in the lateral decubitus position (Figure 2.1), creating a curvature in the spine and thus opening up the spaces between the spinous processes of the vertebrae. The anaesthetist then marks the level at which the block is to be performed. Spinal anaesthesia is performed between the L2 and S1 vertebrae. Epidurals, however, can be performed anywhere from the cervical spine down. The higher the placement of the anaesthetic, the higher the level of the

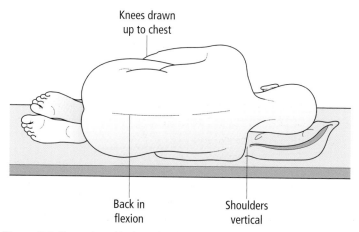

Knees drawn
up to chest

Back in
flexion

Shoulders
vertical

Figure 2.1 Correct positioning of the patient for epidural and spinal anaesthesia

block. An epidural placed at L5, therefore, will produce an anaesthetic effect from that point downwards.

A fully aseptic technique, using gown and gloves, is adopted. The skin is cleaned and anaesthetized. A special-purpose, long 8 cm curved (Huber) blunt tip needle is used. This is inserted through the midline, or by a paramedian approach in the thoracic spine, between two vertebral spinous processes, and is advanced towards the ligamentum flavum. On penetration of this ligament a 'loss of resistance' is experienced and is used to gauge the location of the needle. At this point the needle is located in the extradural space.

If an epidural technique is being followed, a catheter is inserted through the needle at this stage, and repeated doses of local anaesthetic can then be administered to the patient and continued for up to 72 hours postoperatively if required. For spinal anaesthesia the needle is advanced further, penetrating the dural layer and entering the subarachnoid space. A single injection of local anaesthetic is then administered directly into the cerebrospinal fluid (Figure 2.2). The needle and introducer can then be removed and the patient laid in a supine position.

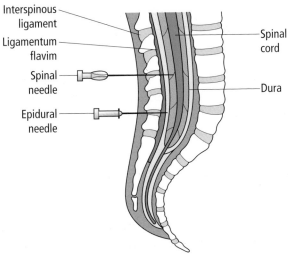

Interspinous ligament
Ligamentum flavim
Spinal needle
Epidural needle
Spinal cord
Dura

Figure 2.2 The course of the needle in epidural and spinal anaesthesia

Peripheral blocks

Peripheral blockade is the administration of an anaesthetic to a nerve or group of nerves that lie outside the brain and spinal cord. These blocks can be further subdivided according to the region of the body in which they are sited:

- Head and neck blocks: trigeminal nerve
- Upper limb blocks: brachial plexus
- Truncal blocks: inguinal nerve
- Lower limb block: sciatic nerve.

Peripheral blocks are most frequently used for pain management, or in combination with a general anaesthetic for postoperative pain management.

The technique employed will vary according to the region of the body undergoing blockade but generally involves the following steps:

- Correct positioning of the patient
- Superficial infiltration of local anaesthetic
- Introduction of a short, bevelled needle with a nerve stimulator attached
- Confirmation of the location of the nerve by stimulation and subsequent muscle contraction
- Injection of a local anaesthetic agent around the nerve.

Local anaesthetics

Local anaesthetic agents (such as lidocaine) may also be used to infiltrate the skin and soft tissues to provide anaesthesia around the site of the incision, and often indwelling lines such as arterial and central lines and drains.

ANAESTHETIC PROCEDURES AND EQUIPMENT

There are several practical procedures you can learn easily while on your anaesthetic attachment. These range from simple skills such as intravenous cannulation and the mixing and administration of drugs, to important and life-saving airway skills.

Airway maintenance

There are several techniques that fall into this category, ranging from simple manoeuvres such as the 'head tilt, chin lift', 'jaw thrust' and use of airway adjuncts (such as oropharyngeal or nasopharyngeal airways), to insertion of either laryngeal mask airways (LMA) or endotracheal tubes (ETT) (Figure 2.3).

Laryngeal mask airway

This technique allows for the maintenance of an airway and frees up the anaesthetist's hands:

- The patient's head is extended and their mouth opened.
- The LMA is inserted into the mouth and advanced towards the back of the throat.
- When it can no longer be advanced any further it can be assumed to be in position. A syringe is then used to inflate the LMA cuff with air to secure this position.
- Position of the LMA is confirmed by ventilating the patient and observing for chest wall movement, and by auscultation of the lungs.

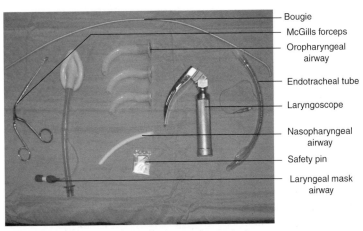

Figure 2.3 Equipment commonly used in the management of a patient's airway

- Tape or a bandage is then used to secure the LMA at the level of the patient's mouth.

> **Key point**
>
> There are many sizes of LMAs. As a rule, women require a size 3, and men a size 4. A size 3 needs 20 mL air, and a size 4 needs 30 mL.

Endotracheal intubation

A cuffed tube in the trachea is used to ensure a definitive airway in an unconscious patient:

- The laryngoscope is inserted into the patient's mouth along the right side of the tongue.
- The curved blade is advanced until it lies at the base of the tongue.
- Gentle force is then applied, pulling the handle of the laryngoscope in the direction of the handle (not as a lever), in order to expose the larynx.
- The tracheal tube is then introduced and passed through the vocal cords.
- Holding the tracheal tube firmly in place, the laryngoscope is then removed and the tracheal tube cuff inflated.
- The position of the tracheal tube is checked by ventilating the patient and observing for chest wall movement, auscultating the lung fields and stomach, and measuring end tidal CO_2.
- If the tube is positioned correctly and successful ventilation is observed, the tube is then fixed in place with tape or a bandage.

> **Key point**
>
> There are many different sizes of ETT. As a rule, women require a size 8, and men a size 9. They should be inserted to approximately 12 cm (to the incisors) in a woman, and 15 cm in a man.

In emergency situations where it has not been possible to starve the patient, a rapid sequence induction (RSI) may be performed. This involves the use of an induction agent, opiate and short-acting muscle relaxant, followed by rapid intubation of the trachea and ventilation. During this procedure it is necessary to apply cricoid pressure to prevent reflux of gastric contents into the trachea. This also gives the operator a better view of the vocal cords.

The anaesthetic machine

The anaesthetic machine is often the focus of the anaesthetist's attention as it monitors the patient's vital signs, ventilation and also the delivery of anaesthetic agents to the patient. Figure 2.4 shows the key features of the anaesthetic machine, but you should ask an anaesthetist to talk you through it.

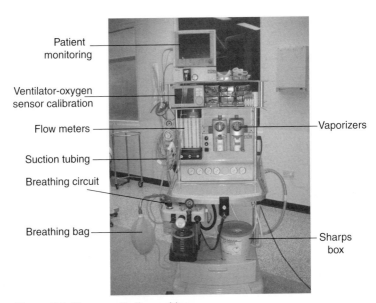

Patient monitoring

Ventilator-oxygen sensor calibration

Flow meters

Suction tubing

Breathing circuit

Breathing bag

Vaporizers

Sharps box

Figure 2.4 The anaesthetic machine

INDUCTION AND MAINTENANCE OF GENERAL ANAESTHESIA

Now that you are familiar with the commonly used drugs, techniques, procedures and equipment, let's outline how a general anaesthetic is delivered.

Pre-anaesthetic checks

Prior to the administration of any anaesthetic the following need to be checked:

- Patient's identity
- Type and site of operation to be performed
- Consent has been obtained
- All jewellery and prostheses have been removed
- The drugs required are drawn up and labelled, double checked for weight and age
- Patient allergies have been considered
- All anaesthetic and resuscitation equipment is available and in good working order
- Emergency drugs are available
- Trained assistant, an operating department practitioner (ODP) is present
- Anaesthetic machine is fully functional.

Consideration should also be given to the patient's preparation for surgery and a set of baseline observations taken:

- Any premedications given
- Patient's preoperative state
- Cardiorespiratory parameters: pulse, blood pressure, respiratory rate, oxygen saturation.

> ## Key point
>
> Pre-anaesthetic checks are extremely important, as surgery cannot proceed unless the patient's safety is assured.

Having completed the checks and observations the patient is now ready to receive their anaesthetic. It is important that from this point on (during induction and throughout monitoring) the familiar ABCDE approach is followed:

- Airway
- Breathing
- Circulation
- Disability
- Exposure.

The general anaesthetic

Induction can be achieved via inhalational or intravenous methods. An intravenous method is now more commonly used:

- Continuous monitoring of the patient is established: pulse oximetry, blood pressure, ECG, pulse rate
- An intravenous cannula is sited in the dorsum of the hand, or in the forearm
- A facemask is placed over the patient's nose and mouth, delivering 100 per cent oxygen (pre-oxygenation reduces the risk of hypoxaemia developing while patient ventilation is being established post induction)
- A test dose of an induction agent (commonly propofol, etomidate or thiopentone) is administered via the cannula
- A potent rapid onset opioid (e.g. fentanyl) is used to attenuate airway reflexes
- The remaining bolus of induction agent is administered through the cannula
- Appropriate airway maintenance techniques are used to establish a patent airway and allow ventilation
- A muscle relaxant is administered through the cannula as indicated (e.g. atracurium)
- An artificial airway device is inserted (e.g. an LMA or ETT)
- The anaesthesia is maintained by using oxygen, a carrier gas (such as nitrous oxide or air) and a volatile agent (for example isoflurane, sevoflurane or desflurane)
- The patient is ventilated as necessary

- The patient is monitored continuously throughout the operation
- Intravenous fluids are administered as appropriate
- Regular opiates with an antiemetic are administered as required to reduce the physiological responses to pain
- On cessation of the procedure, the delivery of anaesthetic agents is stopped and the patient observed for signs of spontaneous ventilation
- Muscle paralysis is reversed if appropriate
- The patient is oxygenated and the airway device is removed
- The patient is transferred from the theatre to the recovery area while still protecting their airway
- Monitoring of the patient continues throughout the recovery period.

Monitoring

An ABCDE approach should be followed. Equipment within theatres provides anaesthetists with immediate and essential information regarding the patient's condition. In addition to this, manual checks are also performed.

Airway

- Observe for tracheal tug, inadequate chest wall movement, reduced movement of the reservoir bag
- Feel for adequate gas flow
- Listen for additional sounds indicating airway compromise (snoring, grunting or stridor).

Breathing

- Look for the colour of the patient (cyanosis), chest wall movements and symmetry, respiratory rate
- Feel for adequate gas flow
- Listen for breath sounds bilaterally
- Measure peripheral oxygen saturation, and end tidal CO_2.

Circulation

- An assessment of circulation involves the measurement of capillary refill time (normal is less than 2 seconds), pulse rate, blood pressure, urine output and monitoring of the ECG trace.

Disability
- Regular blood glucose measurements should be performed in diabetic patients.

Exposure
- The patient's temperature should be closely monitored.

> **Key point**
>
> An ABCDE approach is essential in managing all patients who are acutely unwell, for whatever reason. This includes patients with a decreased conscious level – especially those undergoing general anaesthesia!

THE ANAESTHETIC ROOM

Although the anaesthetic room is a confusing place and trainees frequently feel in the way, most are laid out in exactly the same fashion. Figures 2.5 and 2.6 should help you find your way around.

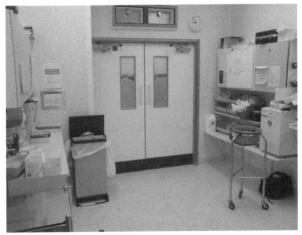

Figure 2.5 Layout of the anaesthetic room

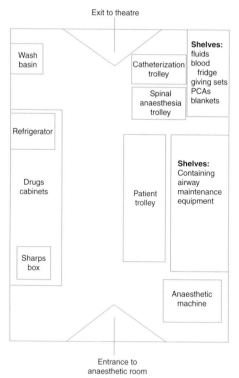

Figure 2.6 Layout of the anaesthetic room

Summary

- Anaesthetic drugs are usually either inhaled or administered intravenously.
- Only a small number of drugs are commonly used, but an understanding of their pharmacology and effects on normal physiology is essential.
- Regional anaesthesia is becoming a more common alternative to general anaesthesia.
- Dealing safely with a patient's airway is an important skill to learn.
- Continuous monitoring of the patient throughout the procedure is critical to safety.

3

THE OPERATING THEATRE

Your first day in theatre may remind you of your first day at school. It is such an unfamiliar environment that it can seem quite daunting or even intimidating. Going to theatre can also be the highlight of your attachment, especially if you have been given the correct preparation before even setting foot in the operating room. It will help you to have some appreciation of the layout, to know who works where, and to have a little grasp of theatre 'etiquette'.

LAYOUT

Theatres are ideally located close to the intensive therapy unit (ITU), high-dependency unit (HDU), emergency department (ED), blood bank, medical imaging and clinical laboratory services. All of these are essential for the efficient and safe management of the surgical patient. Access is usually by swipe card or coded lock. This is to protect the staff and patients, but it is also to separate non-theatre traffic, thereby reducing the possibility of cross-contamination.

Operating theatres are designed with the following in mind:

● Maintaining an aseptic environment

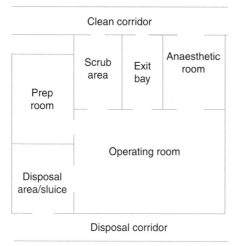

Figure 3.1 Layout of the theatre complex

- Optimizing conditions for surgery – lighting, temperature, acoustic control and air flow
- Ensuring the safety of the patients and staff.

Each theatre has several connected side-rooms, and modern theatres even have two separate corridors. These are divided into four zones, as shown in Figure 3.1.

Protective zone

Think of this as an area where everyday clothing can be worn. It comprises:

- Reception and waiting areas which are connected to the main hospital
- Changing rooms.

Key point

Never leave your valuables in the changing room. Take them with you if a secure locker is not provided.

Clean zone

This area is used to transfer from protective to sterile areas. All staff should be wearing clean 'scrubs' and surgical footwear (conductive so as to avoid static). Spare communal shoes or 'wellies' are usually provided for students. Never borrow the consultant's footwear – even in desperation!

The clean zone consists of:

- Preoperative area
- Anaesthetic induction room
- Scrub area
- Exit bay
- Recovery area
- Staff room
- Storage for all equipment and supplies.

Sterile (aseptic) zone

This is an area in which staff need to be scrubbed and usually sterile gowned in order to complete their tasks. In this zone the conditions are as near to sterile as possible and this is where preparation of the surgical instrument trolley and the operation itself take place. Staff who are 'sterile' are usually gowned in green or blue clothing, and masks covering mouth and nose are worn. Useful rule-of-thumb: avoid touching anyone or anything covered in green (or blue) linen!

The sterile zone includes:

- Areas within the preparation room
- Areas around the operating table, including most of the operating theatre.

Disposal zone

All waste, specimens, linen, exposed instruments (even if not used) should be removed from the sterile zone via the disposal zone. You may for example be taken into these areas to examine an excised specimen. The zone includes:

- A dirty utility area/sluice
- A disposal corridor.

THEATRE DESIGN

The theatre zones are separated by differences in ventilation, temperature and also by different rules. The aim is to have a unidirectional (one-way) flow of air and patients such that there is no contact with pathogens and waste from previous or adjacent patients. Careful design ensures this flow.

Air pressure within the sterile zone is higher than that of the clean zone, hindering the entry of airborne pathogens from outside the sterile zone. To help with this outward flow of air the operating room is cooler (by approx 10°C) than the corridors. The warmer corridor air rises, with the cooler theatre air replacing it.

The air within the theatre is exchanged at least 20 times per hour, ideally with filtered fresh air from outside. Most theatres use a high-efficiency particulate air (HEPA) filter which helps to minimize airborne spread of bacteria and small particles, including skin particles shed by the staff. The pressure, temperature and filtration systems work best in a closed environment, with few people and obstructions to air flow. Because of this it is best to keep the movement of people in and out of theatre to a minimum. Doors are kept shut as much as possible, and never wedged open.

Laminar flow

Some theatres, such as in orthopaedics, require additional measures to ensure isolation. Deep peri-prosthetic infections represent a disaster to the patient and great regret to the surgical team. It has been estimated that in such cases about 98 per cent of infections spread from theatre staff, of which 30 per cent reach the wound via airborne spread. To try to reduce this, laminar air flow systems may be adopted as shown in Figure 3.2. There is usually a strong downward flow of air from above the operating table, sweeping particles away from the operation site and into return ducts below. This system often looks like a box mounted on the ceiling, and there is a line

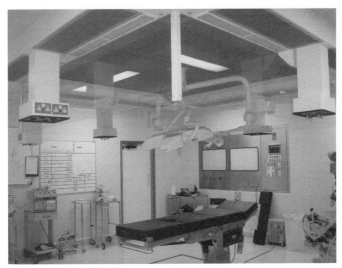

Figure 3.2 The operating theatre and laminar flow system

drawn on the floor. Unless you are scrubbed up and involved in the procedure, keep away from the boxed area so you do not disrupt the flow. Do not cross the line! Laminar flow-equipped operating theatres have been proven to significantly reduce infection in orthopaedic prosthetic implant surgery.

Key point

Do not enter the laminar flow box or cross the line marked on the floor unless you are scrubbed!

Other aspects of theatre design

Other design features of the operating theatre complex include:

● Antistatic walls to prevent dust accumulation
● Seamless water and stain proof walls and floors
● Wide corridors

- Elbow or electronically operated scrub taps
- Sliding doors (preferably electrically operated) to minimize turbulent air flow
- Mobile and easily cleanable equipment
- White, non-reflective walls to prevent alteration to the surgeons' vision and colour perception.

THEATRE STAFF

An operating theatre is both labour-intensive and intense, therefore can feel impersonal. Each theatre, however, usually has a core group of staff you can get to know during your attachment. Everyone in the clean and sterile zones of the theatre complex will be wearing scrubs so it can be difficult to know each person's role, and whom to ask for help. Don't be afraid to ask – but choose your moment. It will help if you can quickly learn the local hat colour code. Colours used may represent both craft and seniority. Learn also to read security (name) badges at a distance – these are compulsory to wear nowadays.

> ### Key point
>
> If you're not sure who somebody is in theatre, don't be afraid to ask. Likewise, always wear your ID badge high on your scrubs so people know who you are, not down at waist level!

Theatre personnel

Surgeon

Usually a consultant, specialist registrar (SpR), senior house officer (SHO) or, post-Modernising Medical Careers (MMC), a specialist trainee (StR), the operating surgeon actually performs the operation and is responsible for its overall success. When a trainee operates, there will usually be supervision, either scrubbed in or nearby depending on the trainee's seniority and experience. The operating surgeon may be helped by one or two assistants, and the roles might be rotated during some procedures. You may be invited to scrub and assist with minor procedures, in which case follow all instructions to the letter!

Up-to-date information on how surgeons work can be found on the web at: www.rcseng.ac.uk and on surgical training at: www.iscp.ac.uk.

Anaesthetist

The anaesthetist is more than just the doctor who delivers the anaesthetic! Anaesthetists have the skills and expertise to deal with many acute clinical emergencies. In addition they also provide acute and chronic pain management services, and deliver intensive and high-dependency care.

More information on anaesthetists and anaesthetic training can be found on the web at: www.rcoa.ac.uk.

Theatre manager

The theatre manager oversees the administrative and practical issues for theatres, and is usually from a clinical background.

Theatre nurse

Also referred to as scrub nurses, these personnel are nursing staff who are trained to scrub and assist the surgeon. Some may be trained to assist as anaesthetic nurses.

More information is available via the web: www.natn.org.uk.

Operating department practitioners (ODPs) (previously ODAs)

Operating department practitioners are staff qualified to assist the anaesthetist during induction of the anaesthetic, assist the surgeon during the procedure and help monitor the patient during recovery.

Nowadays, ODPs and theatre nurses are often referred to as theatre practitioners, recognizing the substantial overlap in their roles.

More information is available via the web: www.aodp.org.

Porters

Porters have an essential role in transporting the patients, specimens and often urgent blood supplies. They are vital to keeping the list running on time, and good porters also play a role in reassuring patients as they are transported from the wards.

Auxiliaries

These are members of the nursing staff who assist in the general running of the theatre and patient throughput. They often circulate between theatres as required, and hence are often referred to (along with nursing staff and ODPs) as 'circulating staff'.

Trainees

Trainees in all theatre disciplines have an active learning role. They usually wear a different coloured surgical hat (such as bright pink!) identifying them as someone to teach and preventing them from receiving any unsupervised patient responsibility.

THEATRE ETIQUETTE

There are lots of unwritten rules that will help you make the most of your surgical attachment and keep you out of trouble. These do vary however depending on the individual theatre, surgeon or specialty. Here is a helpful guide:

● Contact your surgeon's secretary at least the day before the operating list so you know what procedures are being performed and at what time. This means you can prepare for at least some of the basic questions you may be asked, and it also means you get there at the right time. If possible, see the patient and read their notes beforehand. Knowing the patient's history will not only help you to learn the important points about the procedure, but will also go down well with your supervisors.

- You may be expected to attend the pre-op ward round. If this is the case then arrive early on the appropriate ward and check with the surgical or ward team that it is still going ahead. These ward rounds are very variable by nature and are subject to change at the last minute.
- If you have not been shown around, scout out theatres prior to your first list. Arrive at theatres early with your ID badge visible and dressed as you would for any clinical day. Do not arrive in jeans, as your team may invite you to join the post-op ward round.
- Once in theatres introduce yourself to the nearest member of staff and ask their advice as to who you should introduce yourself to and also where to find, or indeed how to get into, the changing rooms.
- You will need to change into a set of scrubs, sometimes called 'greens' or 'blues'. These will be folded on shelves in size order. Purists will argue you should put the top on first so any skin shed or hair lost when taking off your clothes or putting on the scrubs will not fall onto your fresh scrubs.
- Do not fall prey to the prank of being told that you must strip completely before donning scrubs! Underwear and socks (clean of course) are permitted – theatre air flow can leave you feeling cold. Remember, however, that paediatric theatres are kept warm, especially if a neonate is on the list, and you will need to dress cooler.
- You need to choose a pair of shoes or boots to wear. These are often difficult to find. Sometimes they will be in a box for you to pair up, sometimes you will have to find them around the changing rooms, or even sign a pair out. A valuable tip is not to take your consultant's shoes, usually marked with their name or initials. At times it will be unavoidable to use marked shoes, but pick them carefully. It is best to wear socks with the shoes or, especially if you have big feet, consider purchasing your own (www.mortonmedical.co.uk).

> **Key point**
>
> You can wear a clean T-shirt or vest under your scrubs if you are cold. Bear in mind this may make you too hot if you scrub in for the operation.

- Before leaving the changing room, put on an appropriate surgical hat. These will be labelled on the box and will often be different colours for different members of staff. Orthopaedic theatres will expect you to wear a complete balaclava-type hat for infection control purposes.
- Unless you have a locker, do not leave valuables in the changing room. Once fully dressed, leave the changing rooms with your ID badge visible and ask for/find the appropriate theatre.
- Do go and check how previous patients are faring in recovery. If there is nothing else to do then ensure that you have some (educational) reading material with you.
- Some teams may organize for you to come down with a patient, watch them being checked into the waiting area, anaesthetized, operated upon and recovered, and then ask you to accompany the patient back to the ward. This helps you to appreciate the patient's journey, and if it is not organized for you, try to negotiate this. If you also clerk the patient concerned, they will greatly value seeing a friendly and familiar face before and after their operation. This is an easy way of becoming 'involved' in the surgical experience and you will find such unofficial escort duties very rewarding.
- Enter the individual theatre via the scrub room and again introduce yourself. If an operation is under way either wait outside or wait for an appropriate time to ask a member of staff, such as the theatre practitioner, for advice.
- When appropriate, introduce yourself to the surgeon, anaesthetist, scrub nurse and ODPs. Ask the anaesthetist if you can go in the anaesthetic room. Observing an induction

is not only interesting but an essential part of your training. Do not enter the anaesthetic room if an induction is already in progress as this can frighten the patient and irritate the consultant.

● In the anaesthetic room try to be as involved as you can without disrupting the normal routine. This will usually include helping to bring the patient into the anaesthetic room and talking to them. You may also be allowed to place the IV cannula. Anaesthetists are usually the best people to learn this technique from as they are used to cannulating very difficult veins. You may also be asked to help bring the patient into the operating room and join in transferring the patient onto the operating table.

● Ask if you can scrub in (see Chapter 4). If in doubt about how to scrub up, ask if someone can watch you for your first couple of times. A scrub nurse is almost always a better teacher rather than a surgeon! Remember to thank them afterwards and ask how you are doing – are there any things you need to pay more attention to?

Once scrubbed you are now ready to assist (see Chapter 6).

● If at any time you feel faint or uncomfortable let the surgeon know and step away from the table. Someone will come and stand behind you. If you can, fall away from the operating

---

Key point

Feeling faint in such a strange and stressful environment is physiologically normal! Don't be embarrassed, as almost everybody working in theatres will have done so themselves before at some stage in their career. Standing for long periods of time, seeing 'gory' anatomy for the first time, or lack of a decent breakfast are likely reasons, none of which mean you are unsuitable for working as a surgeon.

site as this will avoid contaminating the surgeon or patient and will minimize the potential for needlestick injuries.

- During a procedure it is best not to ask too many questions unless encouraged by your consultant. This is often difficult to gauge; try to pick a time when things are going well and the theatre seems quiet.
- When the procedure is over you should be available to help transfer the patient onto the bed and offer to help push the bed back to recovery. This will also be useful as you will see the handover to the recovery team.
- Between procedures the surgical team may go to the staffroom for a coffee or lunch etc. You should accompany them unless told otherwise. There may be a coffee vending machine or a kitchen with a kettle. If this is the case be aware that you may be expected to make a small contribution.

Key point

It is surprisingly easy to become dehydrated in the specially created atmosphere of the operating room. Make sure you drink plenty of water when you can and have a good breakfast. Remember to empty your bladder if you are scrubbing for a long procedure.

- If staying for a whole day, consider bringing a packed lunch as it will be much easier than changing and coming back, especially if time is restricted.
- At the end of your day collect any appropriate signatures for your logbook and always remember to thank the whole team.
- Check that you have taken all of your valuables and textbooks with you.

Summary

- The operating theatre is designed to ensure patient safety, and specifically to minimize infection risk. Follow the rules and play your part!
- A number of key personnel are involved in the functioning of the operating theatre. Familiarize yourself with them.
- There are a number of written and unwritten rules with which you need to become familiar as early as possible in your attachment.

4

SCRUBBING UP

Scrubbing up refers to hand and forearm cleansing which, together with donning a surgical gown, permits surgery to take place in as sterile an environment as possible. This is especially relevant now that antibiotic resistance amongst microorganisms has become potentially life-threatening. Anyone coming into contact with sterile instruments or the patient during the operation must be properly scrubbed up. This usually includes the surgeon, their assistant(s) and the scrub nurse. You may be included in the scrub team as a student; it is vital that you play your part and your teachers should ensure that you are trained and supervised adequately to achieve this.

Certain preparation is necessary before scrubbing up can be performed:

- Nails must be trimmed and kept visibly clean. Long, fashionable nails are not an option!
- Remove all jewellery and watches, including rings
- Make sure you are wearing a surgical hat (of the correct colour)
- Put on a mask before scrubbing – this is not sterile
- Have an opened gown pack and gloves ready on the side, taking care not to touch the inner sterile gown/gloves.

> **Key point**
>
> Ensure you have got at least your hat and mask (and goggles/lead apron if appropriate) on before commencing hand-washing, and follow your hospital's specific protocol.

HAND-WASHING

1. Set the taps to a comfortably warm temperature and a good flow rate.
2. Open the sterile brush and clean under fingernails with the disposable nail file provided (Figure 4.1).
3. Using your elbow, dispense antiseptic wash such as Betadine or chlorhexidine (see Box 4.1) into the palm of your hand, washing every aspect, including each side and in between each finger (Figure 4.2).

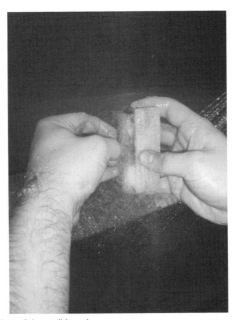

Figure 4.1 Use of the nail brush

Box 4.1   Two surgical antiseptic agents compared

Chlorhexidine gluconate

Advantages

- Rapid antibacterial action
- Prolonged action
- Only rarely problems with allergy.

Disadvantages

- Inactive against bacterial spores
- Variable antifungal and antiviral activity
- Some skin sensitivity.

Povidone iodine (Betadine)

Advantages

- Better at killing most organisms – bactericidal, viricidal, and fungicidal properties.

Disadvantages

- Poor prolonged action
- Higher risk of skin sensitivity (allergic) reactions.

---

4. Re-dispense antiseptic wash and work the lather from the hands towards the elbow, covering each surface of the arm. Repeat for the other arm.

There is debate about the advantages and disadvantages of scrubbing with a brush. These include potentially increasing irritancy, as well as actually increasing infection risks as prolonged skin-brushing may adversely draw organisms from deep pores onto the surface of the skin. The optimum length of scrub time is hard to determine, varies from person to person and there is some evidence even for seasonal changes. The most commonly accepted advice is to use the brush only for fingernails, and to wash the hands and forearm vigorously for several minutes in total. If in doubt check the local protocol.

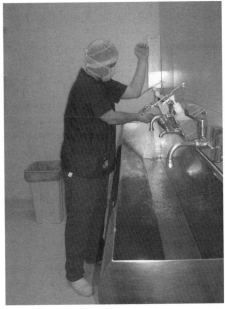

Figure 4.2 Dispensing soap/antibacterial agents from the dispenser

5. When finished with the brush, drop it into the sink unless told otherwise.
6. Keeping your hands above your elbows, bring your fingertips together and rinse progressively from the fingertips down towards the elbow. Rinse one hand and arm at a time (Figure 4.3).
7. Repeat steps 3–6 for a further two cycles. If at any time you accidentally touch the taps or another person or object, you

---

Key point

When washing hands, remember this sequence for both hands: palm to palm, fingertips to palm, interlocking fingers, back of hand, web spaces, thumb. This should take at least 3 minutes!

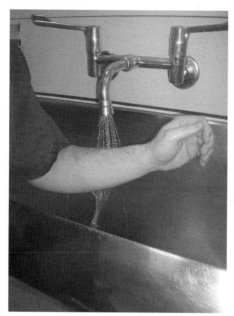

Figure 4.3 Rinse the arms from the hand to the elbow

must start from the beginning or you will be placing the patient at serious risk of infection.

HAND TOWEL TECHNIQUE

Each gown pack contains at least one sterile hand towel. Use one side for the left and the other for the right to minimize spread of infection. As well as making it easier to put them on, drying makes the hands more comfortable in the gloves and, crucially, reduces the bacterial count on the hands.

1. Open up the towel and, as for the scrubbing, dry the opposite hand in a hand-to-elbow direction to minimize contamination (Figure 4.4).
2. Repeat for the other side. Be careful that the towel does not touch anything else, such as the sterile gown.
3. Drop the towel into the scrub bin.

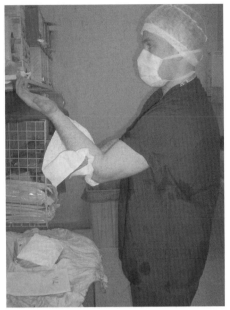

Figure 4.4 Dry the arms from the hand to the elbow

> **Key point**
>
> If there is only one towel in each scrub pack, be sure to use one side for the left hand, and one for the right. Work from the hand to the elbow.

DONNING THE SURGICAL GOWN

The aim of this is to use a technique in which you do not touch the outside of the gown (i.e. a 'closed technique'). To help with this, the gowns are folded with the inside facing you. Some have a barcode or label to help locate the upper inner surface of the gown.

1. Pick up the gown and hold at arm's length. Holding the top of the gown let the remaining part unfold and drop down without touching the floor (Figure 4.5).

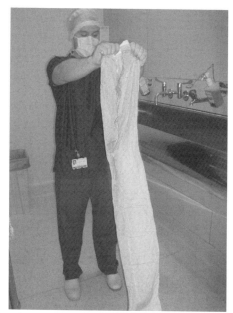

Figure 4.5 Donning the surgical gown

2. Place your arms into the sleeves until they reach the cuffs but no further.
3. Either at this point or after gloving, a nearby member of staff will fasten the waist and neck ties.

> **Key point**
>
> While putting on your surgical gown you need to stand within the sterile field you created upon opening the gown pack.

GLOVING

You can use a closed or open technique for this, but a closed technique will be described here as it is the widely accepted method. Each sterile glove is packaged with the cuff turned down so they can be put on without bare hands touching the outside of the glove. Gloving may require practice, as at first it can be difficult to master.

1. With your hand inside the gown, use a pincer grip (finger and thumb) to pick up the underside of the glove by the turned-down cuff.
2. Place the glove on the palm to be gloved with the fingers pointing towards your elbow. Make sure the thumb of the glove overlies your thumb (still within the gown), as shown in Figure 4.6.
3. Grasp the upperside of the down-turned cuff of the glove between your thumb and finger, and with the opposite hand, say the left hand, fold the cuff around the back of the right hand and over the sleeve. The right hand should now fill the glove. All adjustments for comfort should be made when both gloves are on.
4. Repeat this for the opposite hand (Figure 4.7) and now adjust for comfort.

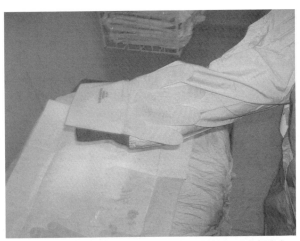

Figure 4.6 Donning the first glove (pinch the underside of the glove, thumb to thumb)

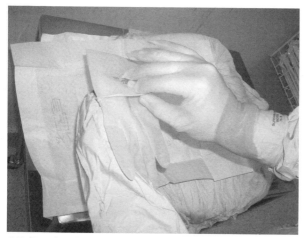

Figure 4.7 Donning the second glove (pinch the upperside of the cuff, and feed over onto the hand whilst keeping hold of the thumb)

Key point

You may be asked what size gloves you require. This often mirrors your shoe size! Glove sizes increase in half sizes from 5½ to 9, the average being 7½ for men and 6½ for women.

CLOSING THE GOWN

The final step in scrubbing up is tying the remaining waist tie on the outside of the gown. This is held in the paper tab on the front of the gown, which connects two ties.

1. Pull the tie labelled for you to hold out of the paper tab, and pass the tab to a nearby member of staff.
2. The paper tab is attached to the long tie, which needs to be wrapped around your back. When asked you will need to turn in the direction indicated to you.
3. Pull the remaining tie from the paper tab the assistant will be holding, which is now not sterile so take care not to touch it.
4. Tie the two ends together at the front of the gown.

If there is no paper tab, you will need to hand the sterile end of the 'long' tie to a scrubbed member of staff and complete the process as above.

Having scrubbed, you can now only touch sterile equipment or drapes (usually green or blue). Your axillae, below the waist and your back are regarded as contaminated areas, so always keep your hands in front of you above waist height. Resist the urge to scratch your nose or adjust your mask; if you do so you will be asked to re-scrub!

Key point

Sometimes before scrubbing you may need to put on special headgear (e.g. in orthopaedics), a lead apron (if X-rays are to be taken in theatre) or protective goggles (e.g. when lasers are being used).

Summary

- Ensure you are correctly dressed before starting to scrub.
- Wash your hands thoroughly and rinse from the hand to the elbow.
- Dry each hand with one side of the hand towel.
- Do not allow the gown to touch any non-sterile areas when donning.
- Practise the closed technique for putting on gloves.
- When scrubbed, touch only sterile (usually blue/green) areas and keep your hands in front of you above waist height.

5

SURGICAL INSTRUMENTS

Students are rarely taught about surgical instruments and the indications for their use. This knowledge is expected to be gained 'on the job'. However, there are hundreds of named instruments across all the surgical specialties and many look remarkably similar. Another confusing factor is that many of the instruments seem to be named after a famous surgeon or institution that, as a student, you have probably never heard of! You will not be expected to know every specialized instrument on the tray when you are assisting, but it is useful to know those most commonly used. This chapter is intended as an introduction to the basics that will aid your understanding of the procedures you will see on your attachments.

Figure 5.1 shows a general surgical tray containing the basic equipment. In addition to this, specialized equipment can be provided depending on the procedure to be performed and the surgeon's preference.

BASIC EQUIPMENT

The contents of a general surgical tray are discussed below:

Waste bag

The purpose of the waste bag is self-explanatory, but remember that some tissue samples will need to be sent for histology and

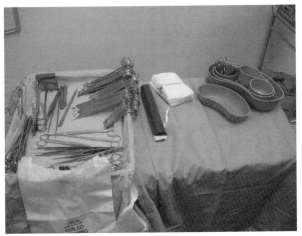

Figure 5.1 A general surgical tray

must not be thrown away. All swabs must also be counted prior to being discarded.

Forceps

There are many different forceps, which can be broadly separated into the types described below (Figure 5.2). They

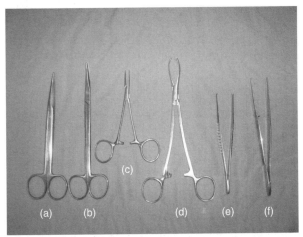

Figure 5.2 Scissors and forceps: (a) Suture scissors, (b) Mayo dissecting scissors, (c) Spencer-Well artery forceps, (d) Babcock intestinal forceps, (e) toothed forceps, (f) McIndoe non-toothed forceps

are held exactly as you would hold a pen, and thus never cross the palm.

Dissecting forceps

These look like big tweezers and can be toothed or non-toothed. Toothed forceps are best for use on the skin as they can grip the dermal layer and avoid the crushing and dragging that the non-toothed forceps would cause when the skin becomes wet. Toothed forceps are generally avoided inside the abdominal cavity due to the risk of bowel perforation or damage to other delicate structures. Examples: DeBakey, McIndoe.

Tissue forceps

These are held like a pair of surgical scissors and have a ratchet mechanism to open and close them. They can be toothed or non-toothed and are used to approximate tissue and remove lumps of tissue after dissection. Examples: Littlewood, Babcock.

Artery forceps

Artery forceps have deeply serrated jaws and control blood loss by crushing the ends of small vessels. They are held like a pair of surgical scissors. The vessels that have been clamped are tied off by the surgeon to prevent bleeding. Example: Spencer-Well.

Scissors

Scissors come in different shapes and sizes designed to complement their function (Figure 5.2). They can have blunt or sharp tips with ends that are straight or curved. The curved scissors allow greater visibility whilst dissecting, whereas straight scissors tend to be used for cutting sutures. Examples: Mayo, McIndoe.

Spongeholders

Spongeholders can be used with a swab (not usually a sponge) to prep the patient before surgery, or as a 'swab on a stick' to keep the anatomical field clear of bleeding during the procedure.

Diathermy wand

Diathermy is a technique used to cut tissue, to coagulate blood and seal off vessels. It is described in detail in Chapter 7.

Retractors

Retractors are used to hold back tissue to expose the area being operated on, and can be hand-held by an assistant or self-retaining. There are many different designs but you will not be required to know them all. Very large retractor systems (e.g. the Omnitract) are fixed to the operating table, and many different shapes of retractor can be secured to them. These systems allow assistants to view and participate in a procedure, rather than simply hanging on to a retractor! As a student you will have plenty of practice using a retractor, and it will help to recognize the names of those most commonly used (Figure 5.3). Examples: Deaver, Langenbeck, Morris.

Scalpel

A scalpel is composed of a blade and a handle. The scalpels used outside of theatre are usually one-piece and disposable, whereas those used in surgery have disposable blades mounted

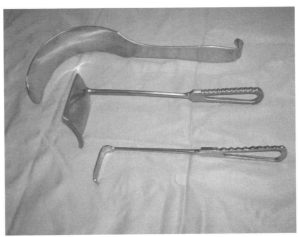

Figure 5.3 Retractors: Deaver (top), Morris (middle), Langenbeck (bottom)

on heavier, well-balanced reusable handles. They are available in different shapes and sizes depending on the type and location of the tissue needing to be cut. The number on the blade indicates its shape.

Swabs

These come in different sizes and are used to mop out fluids and semi-solid contaminants from the operating site. Operating room staff are often seen counting the number of swabs to ensure that each swab is accounted for at the end of the procedure. This is to ensure that swabs are not accidentally left inside a body cavity. In the unlikely event that a swab has been left inside a body cavity, it can be identified on X-ray if it is the type that incorporates a radio-opaque strip (e.g. Raytec).

Towel-clip

Towel clips are used to secure sterile drapes around the patient to keep the working area sterile during the operation. They are blunt to minimize trauma if inadvertently attached to the skin.

Kidney dish

These are more commonly referred to as the receiver, and are used to pass items between the surgeon and scrub nurse that are either difficult or not safe to pass by hand, for example fluids and sharp instruments.

Sterile drapes

Only those scrubbed up are allowed to touch any sterile drape. Usually there will be one scrub nurse or operating department practitioner (ODP) scrubbed up and responsible for the general surgical tray. There should be at least one member of staff available to supply the scrub team with additional material if required.

Quiver

This is an insulated plastic container where the diathermy instruments should be stored when not in use.

Needle holders

Needle holders grasp the suture needle. They look like scissors and have a ratchet mechanism that 'locks off' to prevent the needle from slipping. Example: Mayo.

Key point

There are a lot of surgical instruments, many of which have the same name! Start to develop an appreciation for the different instruments by learning those described here.

SUTURES

A suture is the medical term for a strand of material, commonly known to the lay public as a 'stitch'. Sutures are used to:

● close tissue to aid wound healing,
● ligate (tie off) bleeding vessels, and
● secure medical devices such as a chest tubes or wound drains.

Sutures are available in different sizes, made from synthetic or naturally occurring materials. They may be absorbable or non-absorbable, single-stranded (monofilament) or made of many strands (braided). There could be a needle swaged (attached) to one end, or it may stand alone as a 'tie'. This section aims to provide a clear and concise guide to what can be a confusing topic. By the end of this section you should be able to classify a suture into one of three categories, and describe the advantages and disadvantages of the commonly used sutures.

The ideal suture:

● Is strong enough to provide the support required for the tissue to recover its strength
● Disappears rapidly after recovery of the tissue

- Does not cause an inflammatory response or interfere with wound healing
- Can stretch to accommodate for wound oedema and recoil to enable continuing support of the tissue when the oedema subsides
- Does not become colonized by bacteria or let infection track along its length
- Is easy to handle
- Forms secure knots
- Is inexpensive.

Unfortunately, a suture that matches all these criteria does not exist. The decision of which suture to select depends on its intended use; a surgical abdominal incision, for example, will have different (and multiple) requirements compared with a small laceration on the forearm.

The characteristics of a suture depend on the properties of the material from which it is made, its size and whether it is composed of a single strand (monofilament) or many strands (polyfilament or braided). Box 5.1 lists the various properties of suture material.

Size of the sutures

Sutures are described according to their gauge (diameter). Many years ago the smallest available was assigned a 'gauge 0', with larger sizes represented by increasing numbers. Since sutures were first described in this way, technology has advanced and smaller sutures have been developed. These are described in fractions of gauge 0. For example, 2/0 is half the diameter of 'gauge 0' and 4/0 is a quarter of the size. Metric sizing has not yet become established in the UK but is used widely across Europe. The size of a suture obviously has a bearing on its use (Table 5.1).

Classification system

When asked to describe a suture there are three properties to be considered: natural or synthetic, polyfilament or monofilament, absorbable or non-absorbable.

Box 5.1 Properties of suture material

- *Tensile strength*: A measure of how much force is required to break the suture. The greater the tensile strength, the harder it is to break the suture
- *Knot security*: Good or poor knot security describes the tendency for the knot to slip after being tied
- *Elasticity*: The ability of the suture to stretch and recoil to increasing and decreasing pressures created by the tissues
- *Memory*: The natural tendency of a suture to return to its original shape after being moved
- *Tissue reactivity*: The inflammatory response in the tissues caused by the presence of sutures in the body
- *Handling*: How easy the suture is to manipulate. This is dependent upon other characteristics of the suture. A high amount of memory is associated with poor handling
- *Absorbable or non-absorbable*: Absorbable sutures rapidly degrade within the body. Non-absorbable sutures retain their tensile strength and remain in the body for longer.

Table 5.1 Size of sutures and suitable indication for use

Largest	Indication
1	Abdominal wall closure
0	
2/0	Subcutaneous tissue closure
3/0	
4/0	Wound closure
5/0	
6/0	Cosmetic surgery
7/0	
8/0	Microvascular repair
9/0	
10/0	Ophthalmic surgery

Natural or synthetic

Sutures can be made from natural or synthetic materials. Synthetic sutures have a more predictable absorption time and produce less of an inflammatory response than those made from natural materials. Natural materials, such as silk and catgut, are still used in surgical procedures around the world, although catgut, actually manufactured from sheep or bovine intestine, is no longer used in the UK due to concerns over prion infection risk and unreliable absorption rates in the body.

Polyfilament or monofilament

Polyfilament ('many filaments') sutures are made of strands braided or twisted together. They are easier to handle than single-filament sutures, but carry an increased risk of infection because of the crevices between the strands, which bacteria can colonize. Monofilament sutures are composed of a single strand. They may be more difficult to handle, but are associated with a reduced risk of wound infection.

Absorbable or non-absorbable

Absorbable sutures are degraded inside the body and do not need to be removed. The aim of the absorbable suture is to provide support for the tissue while it regains its strength, and then to dissolve shortly after. Non-absorbable sutures are eventually degraded inside the body but maintain their tensile strength for a lot longer.

All of the information relating to the suture can be found on the outside of the suture packet (Figure 5.4). Box 5.2 describes the most commonly used sutures, including their classifications and their main advantages and disadvantages.

> **Key point**
>
> Braided sutures are easier to handle, but cause more tissue trauma than a smooth monofilament, and carry a theoretically increased risk of infection.

Box 5.2 Common sutures used, their advantages and disadvantages

Polyglactin 910 (Vicryl) – absorbable polyfilament (braided)

Advantages
- Minimal tissue reactivity
- Easy to handle
- Good knot security

Disadvantages
- Braided filament carries an increased risk of infection

Polydioxanone (PDS) – absorbable monofilament

Advantages
- High tensile strength

Disadvantages
- More difficult to handle

Polypropylene (Prolene) – non-absorbable monofilament

Advantages
- High tensile strength
- Low tissue reactivity

Disadvantages
- Reduced knot security (more throws required)

Silk (Perma-hand) – non-absorbable polyfilament (braided)

Advantages
- Very easy handling
- Good knot security

Disadvantages
- Severe tissue reactivity

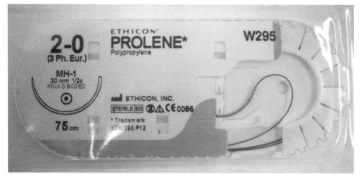

Figure 5.4 A suture packet. All the information relating to the suture and suture needle can be found here

Suture needles

Many types of needle exist within surgical practice. First it may be swaged (with a suture attached), or nonswaged. The body of the needle may be curved or straight. Cutting needles have a triangular cross-section, with the third cutting surface on the inner concave surface of the needle ('surface seeking'). For tissues which are more difficult to penetrate (such as tendons), reverse cutting needles have the third cutting surface on the outer concave surface of the needle ('depth seeking'). Round bodied needles have a sharp tip which flattens to a rectangular/oval cross-section, allowng penetration of tissues without cutting. Finally, for stitching parenchyma, blunt needles are beneficial as again tissue can be dissected without the risk of cutting and subsequent haemorrhage.

Summary

- There are a number of surgical instruments, most of which are named after famous surgeons or institutions. Concentrate on learning about the ones we have presented to you here.
- The ideal suture does not exist!
- Sutures are classified as poly/monofilament, natural/synthetic, absorbable or non-absorbable.
- The size of the suture is expressed as a fraction of gauge 0.

6

THE ART OF SUTURING AND ASSISTING

Suturing is used across all medical specialties and is a skill that every trainee should acquire. In this chapter we will:

- Describe the anatomy and physiology of wound healing
- Refresh the techniques of simple interrupted suturing and one-handed knot tying
- Outline some principles of assisting the surgeon.

WOUND HEALING

The body goes through four phases in response to a penetrating injury: haemostasis, inflammation, proliferation and maturation (Table 6.1). It is important to appreciate that there may be considerable overlap between these phases, as wound healing is a dynamic process. The time-scale for repair depends on the type and site of the wound, and whether there are additional complicating factors such as the presence of co-morbidity.

> **Key point**
>
> The superficial part of a surgical incision, or a penetrating incised wound has three distinct layers: the epidermis, dermis, and subcutaneous tissue.

Table 6.1 The four stages of wound healing

Stage	Name	Length of time	Description
1	Haemostasis	0–1 hours	Blood clot forms
2	Inflammation	<24 hours	Neutrophils phagocytose the blood clot and kill bacteria
		1–5 days	Macrophages aid the elimination of dead tissue by phagocytosis, they also release powerful growth factors and cytokines that stimulate cell proliferation
3	Proliferation	3 days–2/3 weeks	Fibroblasts and myofibroblasts are support cells that proliferate and produce new collagen. Collagen is a family of proteins that in part determines the tensile strength of the tissue
4	Maturation	1 week onwards	Collagen continues to be deposited and simultaneously begins to organize. This process may continue for many months and increases the tensile strength of the wound. The action of myofibroblasts on the actively repairing network of support cells is believed to be responsible for scar contracture early in the maturation phase

ASSESSMENT AND MANAGEMENT OF A WOUND

In the assessment of any wound several questions need to be answered to determine the appropriate management:

● When was the injury sustained? An injury more than 18–24 hours old has a high probability of infection, and ideally should not be closed but left to heal by secondary intention (closing without intervention).

- What was the mechanism of injury? It is important to assess the likelihood of any injury to deeper structures. Injury to deeper structures requires a thorough wound exploration.
- Is it clean or is there debris or necrotic tissue? Prior to closure, the wound must be cleaned, foreign bodies removed and any non-viable tissue debrided. The wound must be thoroughly irrigated (clean tap water will suffice).
- Does it need suturing or can it be closed by another method? This depends on the site of the wound, as well as a number of patient factors such as age.
- Are antibiotics needed? If the wound is likely to be infection prone (for example, animal or human bites), consider leaving the wound to heal by secondary intention and provide antibiotic cover.
- Is a tetanus booster needed? If the patient has had two tetanus boosters in their adult life then they are covered. If there is any doubt, the patient should receive a booster. If they have not received tetanus immunization, they should commence a course of immunization and receive immunoglobulin in the interim if the wound is high risk.

Wound closure

Various methods of wound closure are available. Judgement about which is the best method for a particular case will come with clinical experience.

- *Sutures* are used to help stop bleeding and combat the tension created by surrounding tissues which pull the wound apart. They can be used for large and small wounds alike, although the use of glue or tape may be preferable for the latter.
- *Glue* (Figure 6.1) is suitable for use on small skin wounds that do not require suturing but do need a little extra support to keep the wound edges together. A butyl or octyl form of cyanoacrylate is used, which is less toxic than commercial 'superglue'. Unlike suturing, the application of glue requires neither needles nor the use of anaesthesia.

- *Butterfly sutures* are adhesive strips of tape suitable for use on the skin, sometimes referred to by the tradename Steristrips. They are suitable for minor skin wounds and are also commonly used in surgery to reinforce a subcuticular suturing technique.
- *Staples* provide a very rapid method for closing skin incisions such as a full-length midline incision (Figure 6.1).

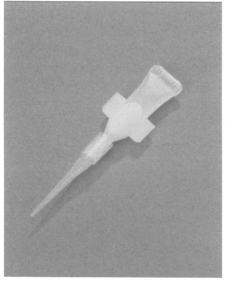

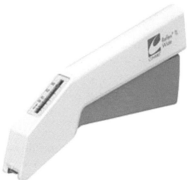

Figure 6.1 Alternatives to sutures for wound closure: skin adhesive applicator (top), stapler (bottom) (Reproduced with permission from Con Med Corporation, www.conmed.com/products_endo_staplers.php June 2007)

They are not as precise as sutures, are more difficult to remove and the resultant scar is sometimes more noticeable.

SUTURING

The first time you suture a wound on a 'real person' will be an exciting yet anxiety-provoking experience, especially if the patient is awake! You will need plenty of practice on a suturing pad and knot-tying rig to become confident with the technique. This section is intended as a revision aid as there is no replacement for practical experience.

To practise suturing you will need:

● Suturing pad
● Suture pack
● Needle holders
● Forceps
● Sharps disposal box.

Hold the forceps with your left hand in the same way you grip a pen. The needle holders and scissors should be held in the right hand with a 'tripod grip'. This is created by placing your thumb in one ring and your ring finger in the second ring. The index finger is the third prong of the tripod and is used to stabilize the body of the instrument. When holding the needle, be sure to grasp the flat section at the swaged (thread) end of the needle (Figure 6.2).

Technique: Suturing and instrument ties

1. Using the forceps, evert the skin on the side of the wound furthest away from you.
2. Whilst everting the skin, insert the needle at 90° to the skin (Figure 6.2).
3. Supinate (make palm face anteriorly) your wrist to advance the needle through the skin and out into the centre of the wound.

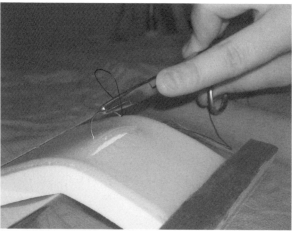

Figure 6.2 Suturing. Hold the needle and approach the skin as shown

4. Reposition the needle, and advance through and out the other side of the wound, remembering to evert the edges of the wound with the forceps (Figure 6.3).
5. Put the forceps down, release the needle from the needle holders and place the needle down to your left hand side.
6. Place the needle holders parallel to and above the 'wound'. Hold the long end of the thread (represented by dark string

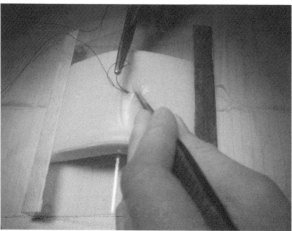

Figure 6.3 Completing the suture. Be sure to evert the wound edges

in Figure 6.4a) with your left hand and loop it once over the mouth of the needle holders.

7. Open the needle holders and grasp the other end of the thread. Next, pull the needle holders towards you and simultaneously pull away from you with your left hand (Figure 6.4b). This creates the first knot and will leave

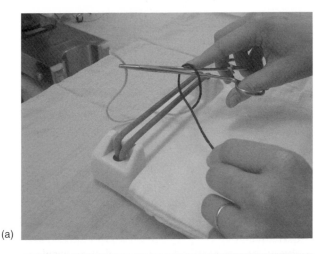

(a)

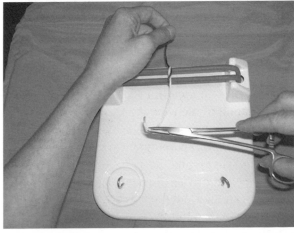

(b)

Figure 6.4 Instrument tie. The technique is illustrated using a length of string to make formation of the knot easier to follow. The dark section represents the end attached to the needle.

the dark end of the thread on the side furthest away from you.

Key point

When properly formed, knots should lie flat!

---

8. Release the thread from the needle holders.
9. Place the needle holders parallel to and above the wound.
10. Hold the dark end of the thread (that has the needle) with your left hand.
11. Loop this twice over the mouth of the needle holders.
12. Open the needle holders and grasp the white end of the thread on the opposite side.
13. Pull towards you with your left hand and simultaneously pull away from you with your needle holders. This creates the second knot, which should lie flat on the first.
14. Repeat steps 8–13 for a third knot. The number of 'half hitches' depends on the suture material (see below). Three is the minimum required using braided material.
15. Cut the sutures leaving at least 5 mm in length to allow for easy removal.

Tips for good results

- *Achieve good skin apposition*. This is the result of good approximation of the wound edges, bringing the two edges of the wound together to create the best possible scar.
- *Take equal 'bites'*. Incorporate equal amounts of tissue from each side of the wound. Be symmetrical!
- *Aim to create a tension-free environment for wound healing*. Keep the wound tension-free by refraining from tying the knots too tightly, which could cause tissue necrosis. Remember that the idea of suturing is to create a tension-free environment for the tissues to meet themselves.

- *Evert the edges of the wound when suturing.* Scars form not only in the horizontal plane but also in the vertical plane. For this reason the edges should be everted (turned out) so that when the tissue does contract during scar formation, the wound does not become indrawn.
- *Do not leave the knots overlying the wound.* The knots may act as a direct irritant or as a source of infection, and should therefore be pulled to one side. This also aids their subsequent removal.

TYING SURGICAL KNOTS

Being able to tie a secure knot is an essential skill, which any budding surgeon must master! Most trainees will have the opportunity to suture and tie knots at some point early in their career. It is a good idea to have some prior knowledge of how to perform these skills, as they are rarely taught from scratch.

The technique is difficult to master and requires a lot of practice. It is important to learn the steps slowly and thoroughly: there is no point in being able to tie a knot quickly if it is not secure! Speed will come with practice.

The one-handed reef knot

Although both hands are clearly used to some extent when tying this knot, it is exclusively one hand (usually the left) that forms the loop and completes the knot. The other hand is used to hold the suture outside of the body cavity. The technique is shown in Figures 6.5a–d with dark and light sections of string to help the description.

1. Place your left hand palm down with fingers overlying the dark section of the string and grasp the string in a pincer grip between your index finger and thumb.
2. Supinate (make palm face anteriorly) your left hand, so that your fingers are sandwiched between the dark section of string (Figure 6.5a).

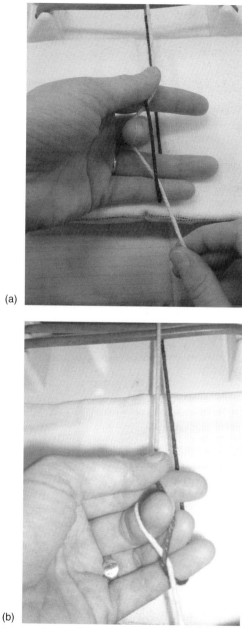

(a)

(b)

Figure 6.5 One-handed reef knot. See text for instructions

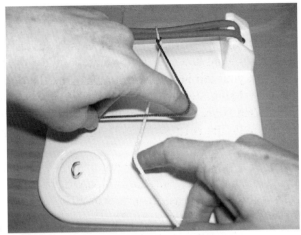

(c)

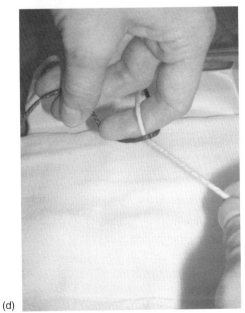

(d)

Figure 6.5 Continued

3. Holding the white string with your right hand between your index finger and thumb, lay your string over the fingers of your left hand so it lies parallel to the dark section of string.

4. Your right hand holds the string taut while the middle finger of your left hand begins to make the first loop of the knot. Using the pad of your middle finger, drag the white string over to the left of the dark string. The nail of your middle finger should now be touching the dark side of the string.

5. From this position you should grasp the dark string between the middle finger and ring finger of your left hand. Do not release this grip. Release the pincer grip between thumb and index finger of your left hand (Figure 6.5b).

6. Pronate (make palm face posteriorly) your left hand, and pull the dark string away from you with your left hand whilst maintaining tension on the white string with your right.

At this stage you should have completed the first flat lying reef knot. The string cannot be slackened therefore a different method is required to tie the second knot.

7. With your left hand palm down (pronated), change your hold on the string to a pincer grip between your middle finger and thumb. Do not let go!

8. Slide your index finger along the string towards the knot. Using your index finger, hook the dark end of the string and move the string approximately 180° anticlockwise to make a right-angled triangle, or mirrored number '4' (Figure 6.5c).

9. Curl the index finger of your left hand under the vertical white string and using the nail of this finger hook it over the horizontal dark end of the string to form the loop. Now clamp the dark end of the string that is emerging through the preformed loop between your middle and index fingers (Figure 6.5d).

10. As the dark string comes through the loop, pull it towards you. At the same time, pull the white end of the string away from you, to ensure the new knot lies square.

How many knots to tie?

The number of knots depends on what type of suture material you are using, and the degree of tension you wish to place on the wound being closed. Knots are held secure by friction, which impairs movement between layers, and this varies with their surface texture. Braided suture typically requires three half-hitch knots, although most surgeons will use more. Smooth monofilament material may require 5–7 knots to achieve security.

Key point

It is vital for the correct formation that when tying a knot your hands swap over. If your left hand starts nearest to you, it must finish away from you, and vice versa.

PRINCIPLES OF ASSISTING THE SURGEON

Assisting the surgeon first requires that you scrub up as described in Chapter 4. Think of your role as providing the surgeon with the best possible view of the operating field – an important responsibility. This will normally consist of holding retractors and other instruments, swabbing tissues and using suction to clear blood from the field. Depending on the procedure, it may also involve offering assistance such as holding the laparoscope and assisting with the use of diathermy.

Try not to get in the way. If you break the concentration of the surgeon you may receive a sharp rebuke! Never take this personally, but be on your guard to avoid repetition. Keep your concentration levels up and think about what might happen next. Being inquisitive can relieve the boredom of assisting during long procedures – but choose your moment. The occurrence of life-threatening haemorrhage or malfunctioning equipment is not the time to chat! The end of a procedure often brings with it a more relaxed atmosphere, as does the subsequent cup of tea in the staffroom, when questions may be asked. Do allow the surgeon to write their operation notes in peace and quiet though.

Key point

Operation notes are always written in the same order – incision, findings, procedure, closure and postoperative instructions.

Some prior knowledge of the procedure to be undertaken will help you to 'second guess' where the surgeon is heading next. A good assistant will be able to identify when a different view is required, and which instruments may be needed next. The scrub nurse generally works two steps ahead of the surgeon, and if you ask them nicely before scrubbing they may be able to pass you the odd cue.

The surgeon may or may not allow you to close – by suturing or otherwise. You are unlikely to be allowed to suture if the team are running behind schedule, or if the case has been particularly difficult. If you keep practising and being proactive in offering to help, suitable opportunities will eventually come your way!

Summary
- There are four stages to wound healing.
- There are a number of alternatives to suturing, including glue, staples and butterfly sutures.
- When suturing, remember to ensure that the knots are secure and lie flat.
- Practise the art of knot tying.
- Assisting the surgeon is essentially about providing them with the best possible view of the operating field.

7

ELECTROSURGERY

Electrosurgery (commonly referred to as diathermy in the UK) is one of the most widely used technical aids to surgery worldwide. Used safely, it offers a range of useful functions including the control of bleeding, the removal and resection of superficial lesions, as well as the cutting and excising of deep tissue.

The advantages of electrosurgery include:

- Reduced overall blood loss
- Increased speed and efficiency
- Improved cosmetic results
- Reduced need for suturing in superficial surgery
- The opportunity for full-thickness excision of skin and subcutaneous lesions with minimal trauma and scarring
- Increased accuracy compared with scalpel and scissors
- Versatility in performing 'shaving' or resection techniques
- Improved haemostasis in excising vascular lesions (e.g. haemangiomas)
- The performance of unique procedures, such as the revolutionary 'large loop excision of transformation zone' (LLETZ) procedure to eliminate localized or *in situ* cervical cancer.

Properly used, electrosurgery is safe, versatile, efficient and enables the surgeon to achieve results otherwise difficult or impossible to achieve. It has revolutionized the way surgeons approach intraoperative problems, as well as considerably decreasing the mortality rate of some operations and invasive procedures.

In this chapter we consider:

● Basic electrical principles
● Electrocautery
● Monopolar electrosurgery
● Bipolar electrosurgery
● Therapeutic effects that can be achieved
● Practical tips for safe and successful electrosurgery.

ELECTRICAL PRINCIPLES

All matter consists of atoms, which in turn consist of protons (positively charged), neutrons (uncharged) and electrons (negatively charged). Let us imagine that we place a finite number of atoms in a row and that all these atoms together make up a solid object in the form of a copper wire. By introducing a force, we can make the orbiting electrons from one atom 'jump' to the next. As electrons leave one atom, they begin to leave the charge of the atom unbalanced, favouring the positive protons. When they arrive onto another atom, they tip the balance the other way, as a result of the excess negative charge. The result of this is that some atoms are now more positively charged, whilst others are more negatively charged, thus creating a net flow of electrons.

In an ideal world we would want this flow to continue unobstructed, however in reality some degree of 'molecular friction' will always exist, in this example it would be proportional to the length and thickness of the wire. This resistance to electron flow produces energy in the form of heat and light, and this key concept is what we harness and manipulate in electrosurgery, as you will later see in the chapter.

> ## Key point
>
> Electrical current will always flow along the path of least resistance.

Electrons always seek to flow towards the electron bank or source that their original atoms are in, thereby completing the circuit. This flow or current can be described as a 'direct current' or 'DC' when the flow is unidirectional around a simple circuit. It can, however, be deliberately alternated in its direction (defined as 'alternating current,' abbreviated to 'AC') over a specified time interval, for example, once every 10 seconds. The frequency of these alterations is measured in cycles per second, or hertz (Hz), so the example above would result in 0.1 Hz.

Considering our theoretical model above, we can clarify some familiar terms:

- *Voltage* is the force (pressure) pushing the current through the conductor (e.g. copper wire) against its resistance. It is measured in volts (V). One volt is required to dissipate 1 watt of power at a current flow of 1 ampere.
- *Current* is the amount of charge (number of electrons) moved in a specified time period. It is measured in amperes or amps (A). One ampere equates to 1 coulomb of charge transferred per second.
- *Circuit* is the uninterrupted pathway formed by a conductor allowing electrons to flow.
- *Resistance* is the opposing force to the electron flow, measured in ohms (Ω). In alternating current circuits it is referred to as 'impedance'.
- *Power* is the energy produced from forcing the current around a circuit, against resistance. It is measured in watts (W). A flow of 1 volt at 1 amp will produce 1 watt of power.

We can define the relationship between these terms mathematically as:

$$\text{Power} = \text{current} \times \text{voltage} \quad (\text{e.g. } 1\,\text{W} = 1\,\text{V} \times 1\,\text{A}) \quad (1)$$

$$\text{Current} = \text{voltage/resistance} \quad (2)$$

Substituting equation (2) into equation (1):

$$\text{Power} = (\text{voltage/resistance}) \times \text{voltage}$$
$$= (\text{voltage} \times \text{voltage})/\text{resistance}$$

$$\text{Power} = \text{voltage}^2/\text{resistance} \quad (\text{e.g. } 1\,\text{W} = 1\,\text{V}^2 \times 1\,\Omega) \quad (3)$$

Electrosurgery is the manipulation of electrical force therapeutically by successfully controlling the variables described above (power, voltage, resistance and current) in addition to their relationship as described by equations (1)–(3). Crucially, electrosurgical units generate alternating current, rather than the DC produced by cardiac defibrillators.

Manipulating the force

When trainees first encounter electrosurgery, they often wonder why patients are not electrocuted. Let us remind ourselves of the electromagnetic spectrum, in particular the section of the spectrum containing radiofrequencies and how these frequencies are used. Table 7.1 lists the frequencies of some commonly used areas of the electromagnetic spectrum. As you can see, the most important fact here is that muscle and nerve stimulation stops at 100 KHz. Any alternating current that operates at a frequency of greater than 100 KHz has much less effect on cells, and in particular will not significantly interfere with nerve and muscle conduction.

Electrosurgical generators operate at frequencies well above this 100 KHz barrier. At such high frequencies, energy transfer becomes very inefficient at any point in a circuit where

Table 7.1 The electromagnetic spectrum

Wavelength	Units	Uses
0	Hz	Direct current
3–30	Hz	Submarine long-range radio
50	Hz	UK household electrical supply
100	*KHz*	*Limit of muscle and nerve stimulation*
150–2000	KHz	AM radio (long and medium wave)
2–30	MHz	Short-wave radio
30–300	MHz	VHF (TV, FM and digital) radio
300–1000	MHz	UHF television
1–30	GHz	Satellite TV, microwave ovens, wireless networking, radar
>300	GHz	Night vision devices

1 GHz = 1000 MHz = 1 000 000 KHz = 1 000 000 000 Hz.

resistance is high, such as the small contact area between the tip of an electrocautery instrument and tissue. This generates heat – hence the term 'diathermy' (Greek: through heat) only at the contact point. A properly applied diathermy contact 'plate' will remain cool so long as it does not peel away and leave a smaller area of contact. All electrocautery instruments have small tips, as a larger contact area would produce less of the heat needed to achieve cautery.

By manipulating the force (that is, voltage) required to 'push' the current, and by altering the way current is generated, several different therapeutic effects can be achieved. 'Pure' high-frequency current at around 2000 V is used to cut by creating steam which explodes cells and tissues. Intermittently pulsed high-frequency current at higher voltages (up to 5000 V) is used to denature proteins both within and outside of cells (including blood), resulting in coagulation. Blended current usefully combines both features, allowing controlled cutting of tissues with some coagulation.

ELECTROCAUTERY

Electrocautery is the simplest way in which we utilize basic electrical principles for therapeutic effect. This could involve destroying tissue or coagulating blood using simple direct current to generate heat in a resistant element at the tip of the instrument. This is now seldom employed, only usually in minor procedures where there is little bleeding and limited cutting of tissues is required. Strictly, electrocautery should not be used to describe any other electrosurgical techniques, the majority of which employ radiofrequency alternating current.

As shown in Figure 7.1, in electrocautery the electrical current alternates backwards and forwards between the two terminals of the electrosurgical unit. The unit is completely isolated from earth. Current passes through the fine looped wire at the tip of the instrument. Contact with tissues completes the circuit, with the electrosurgical generator driving the high-frequency alternating current back and forth. Inefficiency of transmission at the small point of contact between instrument and tissue is lost to heat.

> **Key point**
>
> Simple electrocautery heat generators are now seldom used, except for minor surgical procedures.

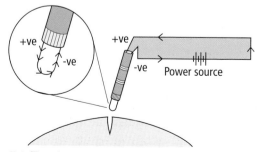

Figure 7.1 The electrocautery circuit

MONOPOLAR ELECTROSURGERY

Monopolar electrosurgery is the most common form used. Monopolar implies the use of a single pole on the electrosurgical instrument, with the patient forming the second pole.

The electrosurgical generator produces the force to drive current back and forth between the 'active' electrode and the patient's body when the two make intermittent contact. The patient is continuously attached to the electrosurgical generator by a large return electrode plate through which the current safely flows when the circuit is completed through tissue contact (Figure 7.2).

As mentioned previously, increasing the current density effectively increases resistance and therefore heat is produced. The active electrode consists of a small tip, and when this small surface area makes contact with tissue, the point of contact offers a high resistance to the current and heating occurs rapidly.

When the circuit is completed, current flows through it. The large conductive pad of the so-called return electrode

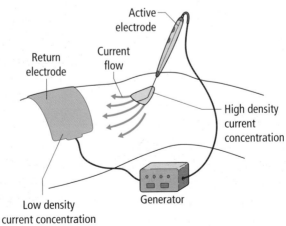

Figure 7.2 The monopolar circuit

has a large surface area, so the current density is low. This ensures that the current produces virtually no heat at this site.

Active electrode

The active electrode may take a variety of forms depending on the type of surgery involved (Figure 7.3). The most common instruments used are forceps and the diathermy 'stick' or wand. A diathermy wand is a pencil-like instrument which can achieve any number of effects using interchangeable tips, such as loops, needles, blades and balls, in addition to disposable and reusable tips used in minimally invasive procedures.

The active electrode can be controlled by either foot pedals or hand switches. These are usually coded as blue for coagulation, and yellow for cutting.

With prolonged use of the same instrument, an eschar of carbonaceous deposit can build up both on the tip and at the surgical site. This has the effect of increasing both resistance

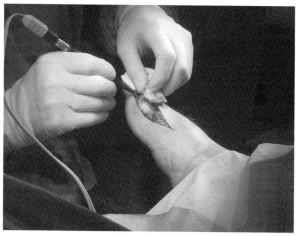

Figure 7.3 The use of electrosurgery equipment in practice (Courtesy of David Edwards)

and heat so must be removed from the active electrode periodically with a special abrasive 'scratch pad'.

Insulated forceps have tips and tops of exposed metal, but their main body is insulated with plastic. By connecting the top to the diathermy, current is allowed to flow through them safely to the tips. This protects against inadvertent flow of current to adjacent tissues. The surgeon is protected by being isolated from the circuit, which in turn is isolated from the earth. It is also possible for an assistant to 'touch' or 'buzz' the top of any metal or other instrument with the diathermy wand in order to create a therapeutic effect. This practice is discouraged, however, as great care is needed when two individuals share control over electrosurgery.

Return electrode

As current flows across the point of contact, the circuit from the generator is completed through the patient via the return electrode (Figure 7.2). The material used for the return 'plate' is most commonly stainless steel coated with a conductive gel to improve contact and therefore reduce resistance and possible heating.

The return electrode should be placed as close as possible to the surgical site and over muscle rather than fat. Muscle conducts much better than fatty, bony or scar tissue. Care should be taken to ensure that the site chosen is not likely to be within an area where fluids pool during surgery, and that the site is kept dry and free of excessive hair. Any unnecessary resistance will generate heat and cause unintentional burning, as will poor plate contact. Most generators monitor contact and will shut down if this happens.

Some pacemakers are susceptible to electrical interference from electrosurgery so if the patient has a pacemaker fitted, it is important to place the return electrode as far away from it as possible. This will direct the current away from the pacemaker

> **Key point**
>
> Positioning the return electrode safely and securely is an
> important job, usually performed either by the nursing staff or
> by operating department practitioners (ODPs).

as it returns to the generator. As always, manufacturer
guidelines should be followed as to which types of pacemaker
are more susceptible.

BIPOLAR ELECTROSURGERY

In bipolar electrosurgery the alternating current passes back
and forth between two poles, with the circuit being completed
at the point of tissue contact. In practice this means that the
current runs down one side of the forceps, through the
patient's tissue, then up the other side of the instrument and
back to the electrosurgical generator. The two sides of the
instrument have to be insulated carefully in view of the high
voltage involved, otherwise current would pass between them
without touching the tissue.

We can see in Figure 7.4 that electrical energy does not
pass through the patient but only across the piece of tissue
between the forceps which completes the circuit. The
distance is small and the arms are close to each other, so
the circuit resistance is low. This means the voltage can
be kept low, achieving the desired effects of haemostasis
without undesired charring of tissue. However, due to the
lower voltages used, bipolar electrosurgery is less effective
on larger bleeds and across bulky areas of tissue. It is
particularly useful in babies and small children, where it
may be safer due to the difficulty of establishing a large
area of plate contact for conventional (monopolar)
electrosurgery. It is also often used when operating on

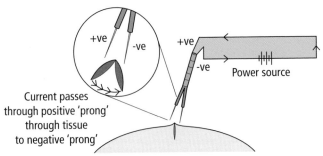

Figure 7.4 Bipolar circuit electrode: current passes from positive 'prong' through tissue to negative 'prong'

> **Key point**
>
> Bipolar surgery is used most effectively in more delicate cases, such as plastics, neurosurgery and gynaecological surgery. It is less well suited to cases which require coagulation of large vessels, or removal of substantial tissue bulk. It is also used in children and when operating on appendages.

appendages (penis, fingers and toes, nose or ears), as the passage of current through an appendage could result in thrombosis of end arteries.

THERAPEUTIC ELECTROSURGICAL EFFECTS

The generator used in electrosurgery allows adjustment of the voltage and therefore power, as well as the waveform of the current being generated. In some cases the wavelength (radiofrequency) can also be selected. By changing settings it is possible to produce a range of tissue effects in addition to those described earlier.

Three common settings or modes are 'cut', 'coagulation' (also known as fulguration) and 'desiccation', each with a

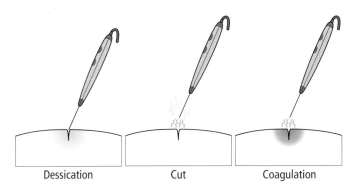

Figure 7.5 Therapeutic effects possible with electrosurgery

distinctive effect on tissue (Figure 7.5). Different tones from the generator may be heard to alert staff to the mode that has been selected.

Cutting

The 'cut' setting is usually represented by a yellow switch or foot pedal and transforms the active electrode into a cutting tool. This effect is created by producing the current as a continuous waveform (i.e. the frequency and length of the cycles each second remain the same). When the active electrode is switched on, the current flows in a continuous form and because of this, lower voltages are required to achieve the required power.

On this setting, the tip of the diathermy should be held just a little above the intended target tissue. This enables the current to flow to the tip and then to the tissue, which generates heat in such a way that cells vaporize without charring. The tip is then advanced along the tissue with minimal pressure and resistance.

The effect on cells is to heat them to the point where all the water contained within is evaporated off, leaving the cells desiccated. The resulting steam ensures that a smooth cutting effect occurs. Some coagulation also occurs, as the blood cells are dried up and all the fluid is vaporized.

The lower voltages lead to minimal heat damage and result in clean cut margins with wound healing comparable to that achieved with a surgical scalpel. The cosmetic result is also very good.

Coagulation (fulguration)

This effect is created by pressing a blue switch or pedal, which sets the generator to coagulation mode. On this setting the radiofrequency waveform produced is further modulated by being switched or interrupted in a square wave pattern.

The intermittent voltage changes result in alternating heating and cooling of tissues. To achieve optimal coagulation, the tip of the active electrode is held slightly above the tissue, allowing the current to spark across. The sparking causes shallow tissue destruction, and therefore can be used in treating skin lesions such as basal cell carcinoma.

Vessel coagulation is best achieved by applying the electrode tip directly onto the tissue whilst simultaneously compressing it, or using a diathermy blade with insulated forceps (as described previously) to grasp the bleeding vessel.

Blended mode

By adjusting the generator to the lower voltage 'cut' setting, and producing a continuous alternating current waveform, the mode can be altered to blend cutting and coagulation effects. Decreasing the voltage will diminish coagulation, whilst higher voltages will increase this. The ratio at which the generator switches between the two waveforms – continuous and interrupted – also creates a specific blend. Higher blend numbers usually signify greater coagulation.

Examples of blended waveforms from generators are given below, where the ratio on:off time is defined as the duty cycle (period of one on-to-off cycle):

- Blend 1 = 50% on, 50% off
- Blend 2 = 40% on, 60% off
- Blend 3 = 25% on, 75% off.

By using a blended mode it is possible to cut whilst coagulating blood at the same time, giving an almost bloodless procedure. It also allows multiple lesions to be treated in rapid succession, with little blood loss and better results.

Desiccation

This tissue effect can be achieved in cutting or coagulation mode, the difference being that the tip of the active electrode makes prolonged contact with the target tissue. Desiccation is used to treat fine telangiectasias or spider haemangiomas.

Key point

Unless tissue desiccation or coagulation in a wet field is required, the tip of the diathermy should be held just away from the target tissue.

PRACTICAL TIPS FOR SUCCESSFUL ELECTROSURGERY

As discussed earlier, many variables can impact on the way the active electrode interacts with its target tissue, including the surface area of tissue contact, current, voltage and type of waveform. All of these can alter the ability of the electrosurgical current to produce heat in an optimally therapeutic way. The following points expand on these principles, and apply them to the practical setting:

- Always ensure you are familiar with the equipment (Figure 7.6).
- Increasing the amount of time the active electrode is used on the target tissue will cause a wider and deeper tissue effect. This may damage adjacent tissues. On the other hand, if this is too short then the desired effect will not be produced.
- The lowest possible power setting should be used to ensure safety, low collateral thermal damage and effective current control. Higher power settings may be needed for obese or emaciated patients than for athletes with increased muscle bulk. The position of the return electrode will also

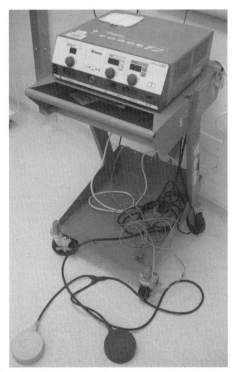

Figure 7.6 The electrosurgery stack

determine resistance and therefore the voltage needed to overcome it. If it is found that increasing voltages are required, the possibility that the return electrode has a poor contact should always be considered.

● If the active electrode tissue contact area is large, a greater voltage will be needed to achieve the same heating effect as a smaller area. Similarly, a clean electrode needs less power then one coated in eschar that impedes the current flow. Only properly designed scratch pads should be used to clean electrodes, as the use of other sharp instruments can leave grooves behind which facilitate the build-up of further eschar.

● Fatty tissue and bone conduct less effectively than muscle. This increases the resistance, requires higher voltage settings and may produce unwanted and potentially dangerous heating effects.

Summary

● Increasing resistance within part of an electrical circuit will lead to dissipation of energy into heat (and light).

● In electrocautery this principle is exploited to heat the tip of an instrument to cauterize.

● Electrosurgery involves using similar instrumentation but the use of high-frequency AC circuits where the small contact area between target tissue and active electrode tip provides high resistance and current density.

● Electrosurgery is used to perform clean tissue cuts, to coagulate, excise or resect tissue, and to seal off bleeding vessels.

● In monopolar electrosurgery, the current is safely passed through the entire patient from active (instrument) to return (plate) electrodes.

● In bipolar electrosurgery only the tissue between the instrument completes the circuit.

● Theoretical and practical training is essential before any surgeon uses electrosurgery equipment. This is provided as part of the mandatory Royal College of Surgeons Basic Surgical Skills Course.

8

MINIMAL ACCESS SURGERY

Minimal access surgery is an umbrella term that encompasses an ever-expanding variety of surgical procedures. In this chapter we will consider those that you will be most likely to encounter and of which you will be expected to have some fundamental knowledge:

- Laparoscopy
- Endosurgery
- Lasers
- Ultrasonic dissection
- Arthroscopy.

LAPAROSCOPY

From its origins in gynaecology, laparoscopic surgery has become increasingly common in general surgery. Since the first laparoscopic cholecystectomy (gallbladder removal) performed in Lyon in 1987, the technique spread rapidly and now the majority of cholecystectomies are carried out laparoscopically. Laparoscopy has both diagnostic and definitive capabilities, making it an ideal instrument for the management of acute appendicitis. The range and volume of procedures being carried out in this way are also rapidly increasing, with some traditionally open procedures, such as a colonic resection, now frequently being carried out laparoscopically. Even complex liver and pancreatic procedures are performed laparoscopically, or with laparoscopic assistance.

Some laparoscopic procedures you may come across include:

- Laparoscopic cholecystectomy ('lap chole')
- Diagnostic laparoscopy (for abdominal or pelvic pain)
- Laparoscopic fundoplication (for gastro-oesophageal reflux)
- Laparoscopic appendicectomy (for diagnosis and treatment)
- Laparoscopic adrenalectomy (for tumour resection)
- Laparoscopic splenectomy (for haematological disease)
- Laparoscopic hernia repair (for inguinal, femoral and incisional hernias)
- Laparoscopic bariatric procedures (for restrictive and malabsorptive procedures).

Modern laparoscopy involves placing a video camera onto a rigid laparoscope to visualize the contents of the abdomen. A bright light source is also required, powered by a halogen or xenon bulb and attached to the laparoscope by an optical fibre cable. The resultant image is passed through a sophisticated computer processor and viewed on a large television monitor (Figure 8.1), so that the surgeon and the operating team can perform surgery using instruments passed through 'ports', which pierce the skin to enter the abdomen.

In order to have a working space to visualize organs, the abdomen must be filled with gas to create a pneumoperitoneum. Initial access is usually achieved by either carefully inserting a spring-loaded Veress needle blindly, close to the umbilicus, or by an open 'cut-down' technique. The patient may be placed in the Trendelenburg position (that is, supine with head lower than pelvis). Initially a little air enters the abdomen and gravity helps bring the abdominal viscera away from the abdominal wall, making damage less likely. Gas, usually carbon dioxide, is insufflated (pumped in) until an intraperitoneal pressure around 10–15 mmHg is reached. This pressure needs to be maintained

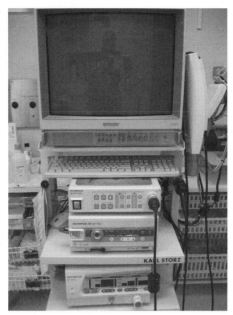

Figure 8.1 The laparoscopic stack

throughout the operation as some of the gas will be absorbed. Carbon dioxide is the preferred gas because it is readily absorbed, excreted by the lungs and is non-combustible.

> ## Key point
>
> A Veress needle is a spring-loaded needle with an outer blunt sheath, designed so that with a decrease in pressure, such as when entering the peritoneal cavity, the sharp needle is withdrawn into a blunt sheath, reducing the risk of perforation.

After Veress needle insufflation and removal of the needle, or creation of a 'cut-down' site, the primary (video) port is inserted through a small skin incision. The port is initially inserted over a trocar (a tapered device that fills the interior of the hollow port), which is withdrawn as soon as the port enters the abdomen and replaced by the laparoscope. The trocar may be blunt or sharp.

Once in place, the laparoscope is passed around the abdomen to exclude any insertion trauma, and then further 'working' ports of 2, 5 or 10 mm can be introduced using the video for guidance, that is under direct visualization. The number and sites of these ports will depend on the procedure, however generally 2–4 ports are needed so that the right number of instruments can be placed in the best positions. Once these are in place, the surgeon can perform the procedure within the expanded peritoneal cavity with relative safety (Figure 8.2). After the procedure, the small port sites can simply be glued, and postoperative pain is usually minimal. Laparoscopy thus allows an increasing number of procedures to be performed as day cases.

There are advantages and disadvantages to doing a procedure laparoscopically compared with traditional open methods (Box 8.1). There has been much publicity about the benefits of

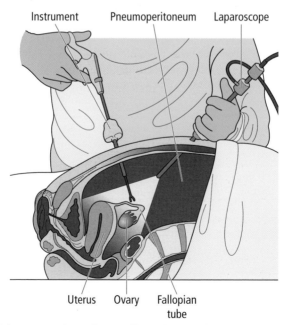

Figure 8.2 Laparoscopic sterilization (Reproduced with permission from Jeremy Brooks-Martin)

Box 8.1 Advantages and disadvantages of laparoscopic surgery

Advantages

- Smaller incisions, less adhesions, smaller scar (incidental improved cosmesis)
- Reduced postoperative pain
- Reduced tissue trauma and blood loss
- Blunting of inflammatory and metabolic disturbance, faster healing
- Fewer complications such as venous thromboembolism (DVT/PE), chest infections, myocardial infarction and strokes
- Improved visualization due to proximity and inherent magnification
- Faster discharge, recovery and return to work and usual activities
- Excellent views for teaching medical students and surgical trainees
- Video recording capability for audit and teaching.

Disadvantages

- Surgeon cannot directly handle the tissue – reduced 'tactile feedback' (only via instruments)
- Longer equipment set-up time, requirement for backup sets
- Technically demanding, more training required
- Instruments pivot on the ports, fixing the angle of approach to tissues
- Ligation and suturing more difficult
- Reduced depth perception from two-dimensional view
- Bleeding easily obscures view
- More expensive operation
- Pooling of blood in the lower body (reverse Trendelenburg position) causing hypotension
- Longer duration of procedures, reduced opportunities for trainees
- Results in less exposure to equivalent open procedures for trainees
- Specific complications of access, pneumoperitoneum and collateral damage from instruments and energy sources.

minimal access, often referred to as 'keyhole surgery', in the lay press. It is important to appreciate that this may be an emotive issue for patients, given a poor appreciation of the risks and benefits by the media. Not all patients are appropriate candidates for a laparoscopic approach and if a patient finds that their surgery cannot be done this way, they may feel very disappointed. Conversely, a few patients fear the risk of serious complications following isolated press reports of alleged 'disasters' with laparoscopy, and may be unaware of the benefits.

The principal 'complication' of laparoscopic procedures is the occasional need to convert to an open approach. The operating surgeon must possess the requisite skills and experience for this, or have an appropriately trained colleague standing by. The reasons for conversion most frequently include uncontrolled haemorrhage, failure to progress due to severe inflammation or fibrosis, distorted or abnormal anatomy, damage to viscera or large vessels, inexperience or an obscured view. Bleeding and perforation can occur with closed and open access. There may also be problems associated with the pneumoperitoneum. Increased intra-abdominal pressure adds pressure to the diaphragm and base of the lungs, causing hypoventilation, hypoxia, pneumothorax or Valsalva effect with reduced cardiac output.

Absorption of carbon dioxide always occurs and can be monitored by the end-tidal monitor on the anaesthetic exhaust circuit. If not dealt with by changing the ventilator settings, hypercarbia may lead to acidosis and cardiac dysrrythmias. Rarely, a carbon dioxide gas embolus can enter the atrium and cause asystole if too high a pressure of pneumoperitoneum is used and a systemic vein is opened. This can occur during laparoscopic cholecystectomy, as the liver surface forming the gallbladder bed is connected to the vena cava by small hepatic venous tributaries. Surgeons and anaesthetists have rapidly learned to work more closely together to avoid and deal with laparoscopic-specific complications.

Electrosurgery within the confined conditions of a laparoscopic approach carries increased hazards of collateral damage, and the smaller diameter of the instruments makes electrical insulation more difficult. This has led to the development of laser, water jet and ultrasonic dissecting equipment, as well as improvements in diathermy equipment such as argon plasma gas coagulation and 'dipolar' sensing electrosurgery.

> ### Key point
>
> Laparoscopy usually refers to an abdominal or pelvic procedure, but the principles have also been applied elsewhere, such as video-assisted thoracoscopic surgery (VATS). Cystoscopy, long established within urology, has also benefited from advances in laparoscopy.

ENDOSURGERY

Endosurgery is a term you are expected to be familiar with. Like 'minimal access', the definition of 'endosurgery' can be confusing as people will use it interchangeably with other terms. Simply put, endosurgery quite literally means surgery associated with endoscopic equipment. As *endo* means 'inside' or 'within' and *scope* means 'to see', an endoscope is any instrument – rigid or flexible – that can be used to look inside the body (Figure 8.3).

You will come across various forms of endoscopy, including bronchoscopy, colonoscopy, sigmoidoscopy, oesophagogastro-duodenoscopy (OGD) and endoscopic retrograde cholangio-pancreatography (ERCP), across your medical and surgical attachments, and it is important to appreciate their diagnostic and therapeutic value. Endoscopes have been engineered to enable procedures to be performed in different parts of the body. To do so they are manufactured in many different sizes and with differing flexibilities. The availability of improved computerized image processing together with the versatility of endoscopes has led to their adoption by almost all surgical specialties. These include gastrointestinal procedures, fetal

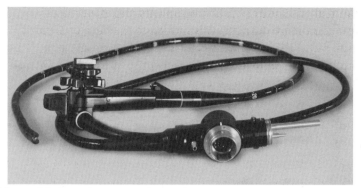

Figure 8.3 An endoscope can be used to access any hollow viscus and allow local surgery

and paediatric surgery, ENT and intracranial neurosurgery, urological procedures and spinal surgery.

Improvements in interventional endoscopy has resulted in the replacement of open surgical procedures by a laparoscopic approach, then later by an endoscopic approach through a natural orifice. Examples include colonoscopic polypectomy, and biliary and duodenal stenting for malignant obstruction.

The latest development in minimally invasive therapy is the fusion of endosurgery with laparoscopic technology. Natural orifice transluminal endoscopic surgery (NOTES) permits the scarless removal of, for example, the gallbladder or appendix, after passage of a flexible endoscope via a transvaginal or transgastric approach. The only scar is internal, after closure of the access point in the vaginal vault or gastric wall.

LASER SURGERY

Laser-assisted surgery has developed significantly since the late 1960s. Public and media opinion would suggest that lasers are used only to treat skin and eye conditions, but the clinical application of lasers is expanding and is currently seen in many surgical specialties, including within endosurgery. It would be beneficial to understand the concept of how lasers work, in what circumstances they are used and which specialists might use them.

Key point

The word 'laser' is an acronym for the underlying process used to produce it: light amplification by stimulated emission of radiation. It was first proposed by Einstein in 1906, but only realized practically in the late 1950s.

Three different types of medical laser are used: CO_2, YAG and KTP, each of which emits energy of differing wavelengths depending on how they are generated. Essentially this happens by exciting electrons from their ground state to an unstable, excited state; these electrons then fall back again towards their ground state, releasing radiation (light). They are stimulated again by optical 'pumping' before reaching the ground state. This continued stimulation helps to propagate a chain reaction of radiation emission which can be used clinically.

Lasers are based on an 'active medium' – the material that exhibits the optical gain – which can be solid, liquid or gas. The various types of laser are named according to their active medium:

● Carbon dioxide (CO_2) laser
● YAG laser based on yttrium, aluminium and garnet
● KTP ('greenlight') laser based on potassium, titanyl and phosphate.

Normal or artificial light contains a mixture of wavelengths, energies and directions of light. Laser energy is emitted as a narrow, coherent, high-energy light beam that is capable of cutting or dissolving tissue and coagulating blood vessels by breaking down bonds in target tissues. The main advantages of lasers are:

● Precise excision of tissue can be achieved
● Both soft tissue (e.g. skin lesions) and hard tissue (e.g. renal stones) can be evaporated
● Minimal damage is caused to the surrounding structures as the thermal energy does not penetrate deeply.

Disadvantages include the danger of strike-past. This occurs where the laser misses the target tissue and results in collateral damage, albeit superficial. Smoke may also be problematic.

The versatility of lasers and the possibility of their use without requiring direct tissue contact means that they can be used in most areas of surgery in addition to dermatology and ophthalmology such as:

● Oncology – palliative debulking of tumours, for example oesophageal and rectal
● ENT – operations on all parts of the airway and oral cavity
● Plastic surgery – reconstructive work
● Urology – urinary tract stones and prostatic hyperplasia.

ULTRASONIC DISSECTION

The first ultrasonic dissector was the Cavitron Ultrasonic Surgical Aspirator (CUSA) (Cavitron Surgical Systems, Inc.), used to shatter tissues whilst preserving blood vessels in brain, spinal cord, liver and pancreatic surgery. Disrupted tissue is aspirated away through an inner tube.

The first implementation of this technology for cutting tissue was the Harmonic Scalpel (Ethicon Endo-Surgery Inc.) (Figure 8.4). This is a scalpel with a difference – it has a blunt blade! Unlike electrosurgery, it does not use heat or direct contact with electricity. Instead it uses ultrasonic frictional forces to generate vibrations at 20–55 kHz. This cuts and coagulates simultaneously, by breaking hydrogen bonds, denaturing

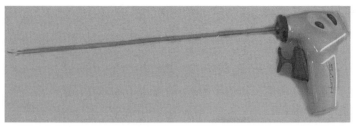

Figure 8.4 Harmonic Scalpel

proteins and sealing off blood vessels. The molecular process is analagous to beating liquid egg-white proteins to form a stiff, semi-solid foam, as when making meringues. It has several advantages over other cutting techniques (Box 8.2), which explains its increasing use, particularly in gastrointestinal

---

Box 8.2   Advantages and disadvantages of ultrasonic dissection technology

Advantages

- Cutting and coagulation take place at lower temperatures compared with electrocautery and lasers. This reduces thermal damage to tissues and subsequent post-op pain, as well as promoting healing and more rapid recovery
- Reduced blood loss, improving visibility and reducing transfusion requirements, especially for patients who are anaemic or those receiving anticoagulant therapy
- Less charring and smoke occurs, affording surgeons much better visibility
- More precise cutting, decreasing the risk of collateral damage
- No electricity is conducted through the patient, eliminating the risk of shock or electrical burn, or interference with pacemakers
- Reduced operating and anaesthetic duration.

Disadvantages

- Higher cost of units compared with electrosurgery
- Need for training for surgeons to become familiar with differences in technique from electrosurgery.

cancer, hepatic, pancreatic and biliary surgery, in both laparoscopic and open procedures. Costs remain greater than for electrosurgery, but are decreasing with increased take-up, and the high costs of litigation for electrosurgical injuries.

ARTHROSCOPY

As the name implies, arthroscopy is a means of looking inside a joint with an endoscope. Originally designed in Japan to diagnose TB in the knee, the technique is now used to visualize the internal anatomy of many joints and also to treat pathology, such as inflammatory and non-inflammatory arthritis, and traumatic injuries such as meniscal tears. Although the joints most accessible to endoscopy are the knee and shoulder, almost any joint can, in theory, be scoped, including the small joints of the hand!

Small incisions (usually two or three) are made in order for the rigid scope and the instruments to be inserted. The scope is connected to a video camera and monitor, enabling the operator to view the interior of the joint at various angles. After the procedure is finished, the port sites are sutured.

The patient will have either a general or a regional anaesthetic for an arthroscopy, as determined by their anaesthetic assessment (see Chapter 1). Depending on the procedure performed, recovery is generally rapid, as evidenced by the widespread application of the technique to treat professional sportsmen and sportswomen.

Key point

A number of instruments can be introduced into the knee joint, including surgical curettes for removal of tissue, surgical graspers, knives, scissors and sutures.

Summary

- The use of minimal access surgery is expanding rapidly.
- A number of procedures previously requiring 'open' approaches can now be performed laparoscopically.
- Laparoscopic procedures require a pneumoperitoneum, and the placement of ports to allow access of instruments.
- Endoscopy allows visual access to various natural orifices and the possibility of intervention via narrow operating channels.
- Electrosurgery is being replaced by laser and ultrasonic technologies.
- Arthroscopy is now used for the diagnosis and treatment of pathology in virtually every joint.

9

HEALTH, SAFETY AND SURGEONS

This chapter could save your life! If not your life, it could save a finger, a foot or an eye. If you're lucky, it will also save you from embarrassing moments such as not knowing which bin to put things in or not knowing which hat to wear.

The 'easy-to-follow tips' listed below give a light approach to this important but often ignored topic. It is important to remember that guidelines are exactly that, and that all health professionals have a legal obligation to promote a safe working environment for patients, themselves and colleagues. This is especially important for surgeons given the small, restricted area they inhabit, filled with specialist equipment and staff of diverse backgrounds – plus students. All theatre staff share this responsibility, regardless of what background or qualifications they have.

Since the Health and Safety at Work Act of 1974, and the Management of Health and Safety at Work Regulations in 1999, employers in the UK have a clear legal obligation to carry out risk assessments. In turn, all health professionals should clearly understand the processes of risk identification and management.

HOW TO AVOID EMBARRASSING YOURSELF

Start with ten top facts:

1. The mantra of an operating theatre is to control infection, maintain a sterile surgical field with safety margins and follow strict aseptic guidelines. Follow these and familiarize yourself with them.
2. Surgical scrubs and footwear must be worn before entering a theatre suite. Typically scrubs are green or blue in colour. Spare clogs for students are usually green or white and are not labelled with a staff member's name!
3. Theatre hats must also be worn at all times. Theatre is not a fashion show, hats must cover all hair, scalp and forehead. Check the colour code for students.
4. The role of surgical masks in reducing infection is controversial but they do protect the wearer from contact with bodily fluids. These should always be handled using strings so not to contaminate the mask itself.
5. Non-sterile gloves may help reduce the volume of fluids and/or blood to which the wearer is exposed. Washing hands between patients and touching equipment, specimens or drapes is good practice.
6. Theatres have ventilation systems to circulate 'dirty air' away from the operating table. Always keep doors closed and always enter through the anaesthetic/scrub room when empty. Theatres are cleaned daily.
7. Equipment is prepared and organized to minimize movement. Respect this – you must not touch anything covered in green or blue sterile drapes if you are not scrubbed up. Always maintain low noise levels – this means no chit chat!
8. Clean and dirty zones are often used for ease of movement of waste and staff. Clinical waste goes in yellow bags, contaminated waste in red bags, dirty linen in white bags, household rubbish in black bags, and re-usable theatre gowns/drapes usually in green bags.

9. Before the start of each operation, there should be a 'stop moment' led by a senior member of theatre staff. Everyone stops what they are doing, and the patient and operation details are read out and verified before starting the procedure.

10. Patients under general anaesthetic are vulnerable and are unable to shout for help. Pay attention and voice any concern you may have if you spot that something is wrong – you may be the only person to do so.

SHARPS AND SWABS

Here are five key points about sharps and swabs:

1. Needles or blades should never be passed directly hand to hand, but should be passed via a 'neutral zone'. This is often achieved by placing them in a kidney dish. Instruments are handed over with the handle pointing towards the recipient (or dish) – never blade first.

2. At strategic points during the operation, the scrub nurse will perform counts of swabs, instruments and sharps, often on a dry-wipe board. This is also repeated at the end and always checked with a second person who also signs the theatre register. The surgeon is informed before closure is complete that the count is correct, and must acknowledge this with a verbal response.

3. Each swab is checked to ensure the radio-opaque strip is intact, so that an X-ray can be requested if it is lost. All items deliberately left inside the patient should be documented.

4. All sharps are a potential source of injury, therefore follow all accepted protocols – avoid manual resheathing of needles and dispose of sharps in the yellow plastic sharp bins.

5. Needles and blades must be mounted on proper holders and never used with fingers. In the event of a sharps or needlestick injury, it should be managed and reported to

occupational health according to local policy. Theatre staff will advise you and be sympathetic – most will have gone through the process themselves.

SPECIAL HAZARDS

Electrosurgery

Electrosurgery and its risks were discussed in Chapter 7. Here we will emphasize a few important specific safety measures to protect patients and staff.

You will remember that a loose connection may mean that any part of a patient's body has the potential to act as a 'return' electrode. This can result in quite serious burns, but because the patient is under anaesthetic he or she is unable report the burning sensation. Patient contact monitoring is used to detect any such problems. It works by using return electrodes split side by side, checking the quality and quantity of contact between them using a small monitoring current. This detects any changes that occur in resistance which could result in the patient receiving a return electrode plate burn. If a problem is detected, the system is deactivated and an alarm generated to alert staff.

The other areas of concern for electrical burns include inadvertent contact with and between metal instruments, insulation failure in re-usable instruments, and capacitive coupling (this can occur when insulated metal instruments are placed inside metal ports during laparoscopic procedures).

The safe care of patients is the highest priority during electrosurgical procedures. Outlined below are specific measures to ensure patient safety, as well as that of all persons present during the perioperative period.

Preoperative
● Surgeons must understand, familiarize themselves with, prepare and check all electrosurgical equipment prior to

use, including reading manufacturers' guidelines and advice

● All flammable materials should be avoided during procedures, including the drugs administered to the patient (such as inhalational anaesthetics)

● Theatre nurses must always document the model and serial number of the electrosurgical generator used in patient records, as well as the exact anatomical pad position and the condition of the skin to be covered.

Intraoperative

● Care should be taken with alcohol-based preparations, ensuring the skin is dry before surgery begins

● The lowest possible power settings should be used

● Intermittent activation of the system is safer than prolonged activation

● Care should be taken with conductive (metallic) objects close to the active electrode

● The active electrode must be maintained free of eschar and the return electrode pad kept in good working order throughout the procedure

● The active electrode should be removed from the patient and surgical field when not in use, and placed in the insulated, protective 'quiver'

● Fluids and liquids should never be stored or placed in the vicinity of the active electrode.

Postoperative

● At the end of a procedure the equipment and generator must be turned off correctly

● The return electrode should be checked, together with the underlying skin and pad surface, seeking evidence of injury

● The active electrode, generator, pedals and cords should all be properly checked and cleaned (although the majority are now disposable – for single patient use).

Surgical smoke, volatile liquids and fire

Research has shown that surgical smoke resulting from electrosurgery or laser surgery contains toxic and carcinogenic elements. These may enter the patient's bloodstream and produce met- or carboxy-haemoglobin, which can be hazardous to the patient. These toxic gases can also lead to fatigue, nausea and headaches in staff. For this reason, exhaust suction is usually applied in the close vicinity of electrosurgical instruments to remove these harmful gases, usually in the form of a 'sucker' tube. Do not suck when there is bleeding or other fluid in the surgeon's way.

Care should be taken when volatile liquids are employed. A common example is methyl methacrylate, which forms the bone cement in orthopaedic joint implant surgery. The vapour that results is highly irritant to the eyes and respiratory passages, and it can also permeate soft contact lenses, which should not be worn.

In the event of a fire, the alarm should be raised and local procedures followed. Familiarize yourself with these prior to entering a new building or complex. Theatres usually have sealed fire doors to enable procedures to continue.

Laser surgery

During laser surgery it is important that both staff and patients wear eye protection. If the beam gets transmitted or even reflected into the eye it can burn the retina, leaving a blind spot, or even burn the optic disc, resulting in permanent blindness. The cornea, lens, aqueous and vitreous humours are also at risk.

The skin can also be affected by laser radiation, causing a burning sensation. This must also be shielded – and as with the goggles, the skin of the anaesthetized patient may also have to be protected.

When lasers are in use, it is essential that doors and windows are closed and locked, with enough warning signs outside to alert and protect staff outside theatre.

X-RAYS

During your surgical attachment you may encounter the use of X-rays in the operating theatre. X-rays are used for a variety of procedures in several specialties such as orthopaedics, urology, obstetrics and gynaecology, and certain sub-specialties within general surgery.

A mobile C-arm image intensifier is generally used in theatre, which produces both still and real-time images. Depending on the requirements of the specific case, the screening time (length of time the radiographer activates the radiation exposure) can vary widely. In orthopaedics, for example, a simple manipulation under anaesthesia (MUA) requires very little screening, about 0.2 minutes on average. However, a femoral nailing procedure is more complex, with an average screening time of 1.8 minutes. The longer the screening time the higher the potential radiation exposure to patients and staff.

You may wonder why this is important to you, but under the Ionising Radiation (Medical Exposure) Regulations (IRMER) 2000 legislation, the radiographer has a duty of care to protect patients and staff by ensuring that radiation doses are kept as low as reasonably practicable. Although it is the responsibility of the radiographer to ensure that there are systems of work in place to minimize radiation doses in theatre, there are a number of things that you can do to ensure that you are protected during a procedure requiring the use of ionizing radiation (Box 9.1).

While X-rays are being produced, only essential personnel should be present in the theatre and they should be protected using a lead gown and thyroid shield. Do talk to the radiographer when you and they are able to do so – they will

---

Box 9.1   Do's and don'ts of radiation safety

Do's

- Wear a lead gown and remember to put it on before you scrub up
- Ensure that it is the correct length (i.e. covers down to mid-thigh at least)
- Wear a thyroid shield if available
- Always replace the lead gown on the hangers provided – if they are folded the lead particles will crack and no longer provide protection
- Observe the images produced to help your learning and understanding of the procedure, and also improve your anatomy.

Don'ts

- Never enter the operating theatre when the controlled area light (found above the doors to theatre) is flashing, unless you are protected with a lead gown
- Do not put your hand in the primary beam when you are assisting
- Do not stand in the primary beam when the C-arm is in the lateral position (if in doubt ask the radiographer where it is safest to stand)
- Do not touch the C-arm. Note that part of it may be covered with a sterile sheet (which may be clear plastic rather than green or blue).

---

be pleased to tell you about how they balance safety with the delivery of precise imaging.

Some hospitals may provide thermoluminescent dosimeter (TLD) badges, which will record any radiation you are exposed to. If your hospital provides them you should wear them as they may highlight areas of bad practice.

INFECTIOUS DISEASES

The incidence of infectious diseases (e.g. HIV, hepatitis B and C) is rapidly increasing. In addition to this, there are increasing problems with hospital-acquired infections including MRSA (methicillin-resistant *Staphylococcus aureus*) and *Clostridium difficile*. Many hospitals undertake 'universal precautions' even in patients not felt to be at high risk of transmissible infection, especially if local incidence is high. In any case, when a patient has a potentially transmissible infection, a number of precautions should be taken:

● The patient should be placed last on that day's list
● All unnecessary equipment and personnel should be removed from theatre
● The patient should be anaesthetized and recovered in the operating theatre where possible
● Extra care should be taken with the scrub routine
● Universal precautions (gown, gloves, facemask and goggles) should always be worn
● Linen should be kept separate and labelled
● Theatre shoes should be covered
● The operating theatre and floors should be cleaned thoroughly with multipurpose detergent between cases.

Summary

● Although a rather dry topic, health and safety is very important.
● An understanding of the basics will stop you looking stupid.
● Be acutely aware of sharps safety and infection control measures.
● Be aware that electrosurgery, laser surgery and X-rays all have specific safety measures in place that you must adhere to.
● If the patient has a potentially transmissible disease you may not be allowed in the theatre. This is for your own safety.

10

YOU AS A TRAINEE

All too often medical students find themselves 'lost among the crowd', 'drifting with the flow' or just 'up the creek without a paddle'. The first time medical students set foot on the wards can be an exciting, nervous and fulfilling experience, but alas, the initial feeling of eagerness and motivation can soon evaporate!

Perhaps you are unsure whether to shadow the busy F1 or go to theatre, as you only end up standing in the corner for 3 hours while the consultant and registrar forget your existence and discuss their golf swings. Perhaps the prospect of endless ward rounds where you are ignored or seemingly told to 'go and look that question up in a book' sap your enthusiasm. Perhaps you are still smarting from the shame you felt when the outpatient sister expelled you because you forgot your white coat or name badge.

This may seem rather a bleak outlook on life during clinicals, and should not represent actual reality nowadays. Nevertheless these events are genuine experiences of the authors over recent years.

The aim of this chapter is to provide guidance and tips on how to obtain the very best from your surgical and anaesthetic attachments, and avoid or deal with experiences such as those described above.

> ## Key point
>
> To get the best out of your time as a student you need to know exactly how to study and how to use your experiences effectively. This is something you are 'expected to know' although it is never formally taught.

MAKING THE MOST OF YOUR ATTACHMENT

It is often the clinical aspect of training that lowers exam marks, as opposed to not having read every medical textbook cover to cover six times! Once you start your clinical training, if you have not noticed thus far, the way you are taught will change as you progress. Long gone are the days of spoon-feeding lectures and endless seminars – you are suddenly thrust onto the wards, theatres and clinics, sometimes with just your consultant's timetable in hand and, if you're very lucky, their secretary's phone number.

At many medical schools, clinical attachments are often well timetabled with teaching programmes and clinic, theatre and on-call rotas provided at induction. It is imperative that mandatory activities are not missed, if only for the obvious reason that these sessions usually do cover essential exam content. Believe us, this cannot 'just be found in textbooks' over the weekend before assessments! If you do miss an activity, for example due to an illness or doctor's appointment, it is courteous to send an apology. Never fabricate excuses; this is unprofessional and if you are discovered you may be asked to attend the Fitness to Practise committee or even reported to the GMC. If a teacher fails to attend after 5 or 10 minutes, do contact your undergraduate education coordinator. There may well be a reason, and your teacher may have made alternative arrangements. If this is not the case, the coordinator will investigate and rearrange the session.

Do not be meek about asking for additional teaching from any member of staff; they will often be delighted to be asked, although many will struggle to find the time to deliver on promises.

Key point

It may sound like a truism, but what you get out of a clinical attachment simply depends on how much energy, time and effort you put in.

Following the advice above, the next bit is up to you. It is common knowledge that in medical school it is easy to just drift along, attending only mandatory sessions and reach finals without anyone batting an eyelid. The outcome, however, is often undesirable. The best medical students get honours not because of medical school teaching methods, but simply because they are fully involved with their team.

These students are often viewed as special beings, with halos around their heads – 'they always get the best teaching', 'must work all through the night' or 'always get lucky when procedures need doing'. We have learnt that none of this is true. The truth is they know their consultant and their consultant knows them. They are on first-name terms with the juniors and the nurses know they can trust them as they saw them being supervised by the F2 the day before, and so on. This is what medical school is all about. And herein lie the consequences. On day one of your F1 job, you are much less likely to look like a loon when you are asked to put a catheter in, to send off bloods, to write in notes on ward rounds or to simply refer someone for an X-ray and chase it up later if you have put in the groundwork.

> **Key point**
>
> It is up to you to make the effort to get to know everyone – not the other way round.

The reality with some medical schools is that traditional apprenticeships on firms are disappearing and students now follow rigid timetabling and rotations every few weeks through different firms. This obviously makes getting involved more difficult, but doing a few on-takes here and there and coming in for the ward rounds and attending meetings will ease the process.

A quick look at our American counterparts perhaps highlights some deficiencies in the British training system. In the US, clinical students are given full responsibility for clerking patients and ordering basic investigations on the wards. They are expected to come up with a differential diagnosis, as well as having results of tests at hand before they are able to present patients. Their clinical years are akin to having a full-time job in an apprenticeship-style arrangement. In the UK it is worth remembering that just because this is not expected of you, it does not mean it is not what you should be doing!

> **Key point**
>
> Getting involved with your team and their daily activities will make you a better doctor in the end. Simple but true.

A TYPICAL DAY

Obviously the 'typical day' described in Box 10.1 is intended only as a rough guide. As you progress through your attachment you will identify your own strengths and weaknesses. It is up to you to attend more clinics or theatre sessions, or carry out more ward work as you see the need.

Box 10.1   A typical day on your surgical attachment

07.45

- Arrive on the ward and help the F1 prepare the notes for your team's 'business ward round' patients.

08.00

- Accompany your team on the daily round. This is usually quick compared to medical rounds – theatre or clinic may be beckoning.
- Take note of interesting patients/conditions with which you are unfamiliar.
- Learn about how to write in the notes, and do so if this is permitted – it is an important skill. Write legibly, sign, time and date each entry, and give a bleep number if you have one. Electronic note systems may be used – obtain a login.

08.40

- Head to theatre with your team and change into scrubs.

09.00

- Speak to the patient and anaesthetist. Ask if you may observe and assist induction of the anaesthetic – an ideal opportunity for cannulation and, if you're lucky, airway skills.
- Look at the X-rays, CT scans, angiograms with the surgeons to enhance your image interpretation skills.
- Enjoy watching and assisting with the operation. Ask questions when safe to do so.

12.00

- All attachments will have a formal teaching programme. This is normally compulsory, and is also a good opportunity to learn about things you haven't yet come across on the wards, in clinic or in theatre.

Box 10.1 (Continued)

13.00

- Teams often have multidisciplinary meetings at lunchtime – a good chance for a 'no such thing as a free lunch' and to learn from the experts. Make notes to look up what you have not understood or were too embarrassed to ask about.

14.00

- Your afternoon may involve attending a specialist clinic or seeing patients on the ward. Opportunities for seeing preoperative patients, practising examinations and taking histories with a 'study buddy' observing you, are numerous. Do socialize but don't just sit in the mess (or the library) all day.

17.30

- OK you could have gone home at 5pm – that's the rule! Almost always the surgical team will do a post-op round to check the patients from theatre that day and to check investigation results on other patients – worth attending.

18.00

- Find out about next day's theatre list and other activities. Head home and if you are car-sharing, chat and reflect with fellow students about what you saw today. Never do this on the bus or train – it's all confidential! You can always wind down at home. Then read up about it – you will remember facts all the more if you can associate them with a patient or operation you have seen.

Medicine is an absorbing but demanding occupation, and will take up a large amount of your life. The experiences you have with people will mature you 'beyond your years'. Use these to deepen your life experience and enjoyment, and excel outside your career. It is vitally important to continue with hobbies and extracurricular activities, just as it is to use your time efficiently during clinical attachments. This will ensure that you are well rounded, which will make you a better doctor.

YOUR ROLE ON THE FIRM

It is important that once placed on your firm, whether for a week or longer, you make every effort to integrate yourself within the team. The key is to be persistent in asking people where your team is, what your consultant is doing and when the ward rounds, clinics and theatre sessions are.

> ### Key point
>
> Do not expect your seniors to come looking or asking to see if you would like to do 'task X'.

Although you may feel like you are stuck 'at the bottom of the food chain', this in actual fact is an enormous advantage! At no other point in your medical career will you have the freedom to pick and choose what you do on the wards, or ask silly questions or receive help, advice and supervision in the way you do when you are still a medical student.

> ### Key point
>
> You have the luxury as a student to ask as many silly questions as you want, or to give the wrong answers to questions you are asked. Do not feel embarrassed; your senior will probably feel pleased that they were able to fill your knowledge gap.

Here's some simple advice to ensure you get the most out of your attachment:

● Turn up to as many ward rounds as you can. They may seem a waste of time initially, but you will find that as your seniors learn that you are interested they will become more inclined to teach and involve you.

- Spend as much time as you can shadowing F1s and offer to help out in whatever tasks they do (including phlebotomy). This is the job you will soon be doing!
- Clerk all new patients who arrive on your wards and hassle your seniors until you find someone to present to.
- Present patients on the ward round, but ensure you have all investigation results at hand. Patient-based teaching on ward rounds cannot be found in books and you will remember the disease and management much better when you can link it to a particular patient.
- Ask your seniors and other students for any patients with interesting histories and physical signs. It does not matter how long they have been in – you will only recognize a murmur or an ileostomy bag in the summative clinical assessment if you have seen one before.
- Get to know the nursing and ancillary staff; they will become an invaluable source in helping you practise lots of practical procedures. Being polite and offering to make or bring them a drink or snack goes a long way to help.
- Get used to how hospital wards and clinics work. Again, on the first day of your new job you do not want to waste time asking people how to fill in request forms, death certificates and how to send off bloods.
- Try to attend handovers between juniors. This will be an invaluable source of information as to who is who on the wards and what stage of their admission they are at.
- Carry a piece of paper with all your firm's patient details on it, and jot down a brief history, examination and investigations with results that have occurred. Keep this up to date and always enquire each day what has happened to them. Remember this information is confidential, and must be disposed of in a confidential waste bin.
- If there is nothing to do (be prepared for this), sit somewhere on the ward with a book. This way you are much more likely to learn opportunistically, such as when reading X-rays and interpreting data and results. This is most useful when using real scenarios.

● The role you will play will largely depend on how much effort and time you are willing to put in. The trick is to become fully integrated within your firm, and only then will you be able to see the most patients, practise the most procedures and receive practical advice and teaching that will prepare you for your job.

HOW TO SOUND IMPRESSIVE

Here are two mnemonics that will make you sound intelligent whenever someone asks you the two most common questions: 'What is disease X?' and 'What causes disease X?'.

What is disease X?

Structure your answer using the mnemonic 'DEEP PIT OF' and you will gain lots of points without even knowing much about disease X, you will look more intelligent and, crucially, you will sound more like a doctor. Feel free to adapt this mnemonic to better suit your learning:

● D – Description of disease (e.g. an inflammatory bowel disorder)
● E – Epidemiology
● E – aEtiology
● P – Pathology
● P – Presentation (includes history and examination findings)
● I – Investigations needed
● T – Treatment of the disease
● O – Outcomes of the disease (e.g. prognosis, treatment success rates, etc.)
● F – Future developments.

What causes disease X?

We have all heard of a surgical sieve, an example is VITAMIN D:

● V – Vascular
● I – Infectious

- T – Traumatic
- A – Autoimmune
- M – Metabolic/endocrine
- I – Iatrogenic/idiopathic
- N – Neoplastic (malignant or benign)
- D – Degenerative

Even simpler than this, most diseases can be split into congenital causes and acquired causes. Again, if you know nothing, in the heat of the moment a mnemonic may jog your memory and save your skin.

Finally, always remember that although a good memory helps, if you understand a disease process you will be able to apply that information to any scenario, which is a far more useful skill. When asked in an exam for five causes of atrial fibrillation, if you understand the physiology you are more likely to remember the disease.

TOP TIPS

In Box 10.2 we have listed some short tips on how to stay one step ahead, look more impressive and make the most out of your opportunities.

Box 10.2   Top tips on how to stay one step ahead

General

- *Introduce yourself personally to consultants and their teams*. This is polite and gives a good first impression.
- *See patients on your own as well as with fellow students*. Get into this habit from day one. Take lots of histories, examine lots of patients and do lots of procedures.
- *Ask lots of questions*. Often if you don't, you will get ignored – this is how you learn.
- *Do as many on-calls as possible*. The best opportunity to get to know your team personally and be the first one to see patients and perform investigations.

Box 10.2 (Continued)

- *Get grilled*. Preferably by a consultant, but a sinister registrar will do. Get used to functioning under pressure to prepare you for tougher times ahead.
- *Dress appropriately*. Consultants wear suits, only doctors get to wear stethoscopes around their necks. Trousers, shirt and tie for the gents. Ladies take care with skirt lengths and plunging neck lines. Don't forget comfortable shoes. With the possible exception of ears, no sites of body piercing should be visible, nor should any tattoos!
- *Look after yourself – eat, sleep and rest well*. Don't be afraid to speak to someone, there is always an impartial supervisor or mentor around and colleagues and friends are always at hand. Ask for help whenever you need it – you are not alone!
- *Do help each other out*. You are not in direct competition with each other at medical school, so get together in groups, practise examinations and share revision resources and tips.
- *Take control of your own curriculum and be persistent*. Only you know what you know and what you don't know, therefore go seek the knowledge you need and organize yourself to do so.
- *Don't be arrogant or shy*. Arrogance will make you hugely unpopular with colleagues and seniors. Being shy will cause you to miss out and fall behind your colleagues.
- *Don't prescribe anything or pretend you're a doctor*. It does happen and has very serious consequences.
- *Never embarrass or show another medical student up*. You are all in the same position and will all face difficult situations, stresses and all make embarrassing mistakes. If it doesn't happen to you today, it might tomorrow, so be sympathetic.
- *Never be late*. If there is one thing that seems to spark an infernal rage of hell in seniors, it is turning up mid-way through a clinic or ward round without good reason.
- *Do not overwork yourself to exhaustion*. When people say they work 24/7, it is not true. You may have an unproductive hour when your colleague is working hard. Don't get stressed, as the opposite will occur – we don't all work the same.

Box 10.2 (Continued)

- *Be aware of medical confidentiality*. It is easy when we see exciting conditions and patients to tell all our friends and families about it, however you are now in a responsible position and patients have the right to medical confidentiality.
- *Don't turn up in the morning still drunk or intoxicated*. Obvious really, but remember if you are still feeling the effects it is irresponsible to be around patients under the influence. Take the morning off. In addition, don't turn up with your breath smelling of last night's beer, curry or garlic-containing meal.

Seniors

- *Never tell nurses or doctors what to do*. A quick way to get out of favour; respect seniors and more qualified people.
- *Never embarrass yourself at the mess parties*. Often a quick way to become known around the hospital for all the wrong reasons. Also 'making a move' on doctors, nurses or other heath professionals is often bad for your health. Patients are always off limits!
- *Never ask seniors to make you a hot drink during clinics or tea breaks*. Again obvious, but it does happen. Offer to do this for them – they are busier than you.

Wards

- *Always introduce yourself to the ward sister*. Life will become easy and nurses will always be happy to point you to interesting patients or help you in your hour of need.
- *Actively seek out doctors*. They will not be looking for you. Doing this will mean more teaching and will improve practical skills (e.g. X-ray and data interpretation, cannulation). This cannot be found in books, and will make your first days as a doctor much easier.
- *Clerk patients and present during ward rounds*. Good practice for the exams, especially as there will be a little bit of pressure on the ward round. Always impresses everyone on your team.
- *Go to lunchtime meetings and journal clubs*. As well as getting lunch and looking impressive, these are excellent times to learn about presentation skills. Often these

Box 10.2 (Continued)

discussions are beyond your curriculum and will push your knowledge towards an honours grade.

- *Foundation year 1 doctors*. Shadow them, badger them and always ask if they need help. This is what you will soon be doing.

- *Ward rounds*. Ask to write in notes on ward rounds if this is allowed. It is a really important skill. Medical rounds tend to be longer and start later than surgical ones. Surgical ones start at 8am. Medical and surgical post take or admission unit rounds can be particularly educational.

Clinics

- *Read up before going to clinic*. It helps if you know a little, otherwise you will end up falling asleep, or worse the doctor will make things very uncomfortable for you. If you have basics upon which to hang things, you will learn more.

- *See patients before they see the doctor if you can*. This makes time go by more quickly and lets you practise your skills. Often you have to ask to do this. Often the doctors are even shocked you asked! Ask if you can go next door and take a patient's history and present it later – it may even help the consultant to run the clinic to time.

- *Refreshments*. How this works is that if you want a drink, ask everyone else if they want one first. Never get someone else to make you one unless they offer. Then leave around 20p per cup; things will turn nasty if you think drinks are free.

Theatre

- *Patients*. Follow patients from clerking, through theatre and postoperatively. If you know nothing about the patient or the operation before going to theatre, be prepared for some uncomfortable questions and a difficult time. Going into theatre unprepared is useless.

- *Introduce yourself*. Make your presence felt or you will get ignored and just stand in a corner for hours. Know who is who in the theatre and keep badgering the surgeon until he or she acknowledges you are there to learn. Obviously if it is a sensitive procedure, restraint and silence are needed for the surgeon to work.

Box 10.2 (Continued)

- *Changing rooms*. Clogs and scrubs are required to enter theatre departments. Memorize the changing room code so when you leave at night you don't get trapped. It is unusual for students to get lockers but ask at reception.
- *Etiquette*. Never steal clogs with names on. Chances are the owner will hunt you down. Separate clogs for students are usually hidden somewhere.
  You must wear a hat – pink ones usually denote untrained personnel, which is you. Sometimes green hats are used for students. Check this to save embarrassment later.
- *Inside theatres*. Theatres are entered through the scrub or prep room. This is to maintain a clean flow of air through the rooms. Unless you are scrubbed up, never touch anything green/blue (sterile). Tuck badges/hair/necklaces in to prevent contaminating surgical fields as you eagerly bend over to have a look.
- *Ask to scrub up*. If you don't, you never will. Most surgeons are very happy to let you get involved, but are often too busy to spend time ensuring a medical student gets a chance to scrub up. A theatre nurse is often the best person to teach you. Remember everyone is eager and happy to teach, but it is up to you to make the first move and get the ball rolling.

THE FOUNDATION PROGRAMME AND SPECIALIST TRAINING

It is an exciting time for a career in medicine! The way doctors train in the UK is being revolutionized with the Modernising Medical Careers (MMC) reforms. In August 2005 the foundation programmes replaced the old pre-registration house officer (PRHO) and first-year senior house officer (SHO) posts.

It is beyond the scope of this chapter to comprehensively outline the new system and the reader is pointed towards the web links at the end for up-to-date sources on the internet.

The overall aim of the foundation programme is to ensure that doctors, whatever speciality, are emergency safe and are able to deal with common chronic conditions and emergencies appropriately. The foundation programme consists of a two-year programme of six different four-month posts, including at least one medical, one surgical and one acute specialty such as accident and emergency medicine or intensive care.

The foundation programme is closely coordinated, providing newly qualified doctors with a set curriculum and protected teaching and training times. Applications for this and, indeed, specialty training (ST) have been made through the Medical Training Application Service (MTAS). The future of selection has not yet been determined.

Trainees progress through the two-year foundation programme before reapplying for ST training (Figure 10.1). ST or speciality training consists of a six- or seven-year programme for which trainees enter a speciality of their choice, for example orthopaedic surgery, general practice, paediatrics, etc. The first level of ST training is named ST1, the second ST2 and so on. Some trainees may take two years to complete one level if assessments are unsatisfactory. To progress successfully, trainees must achieve satisfactory knowledge as well as competency-based skill assessments throughout foundation and ST training. If unsuccessful, trainees may have to enter a non-training post as a staff or associate specialist after their ST2 year, or later at any ST level.

A CAREER IN SURGERY

So how does this affect you? A career in surgery is naturally competitive and places on surgical ST programmes are highly sought after. In order to maximize your chances of getting a place, here are ten pointers:

1. Decide on a career early on. This helps you focus on what things you need to boost your CV and focuses your efforts to maximize your career path. If you can demonstrate longevity of interest, this will score highly in later job interviews.

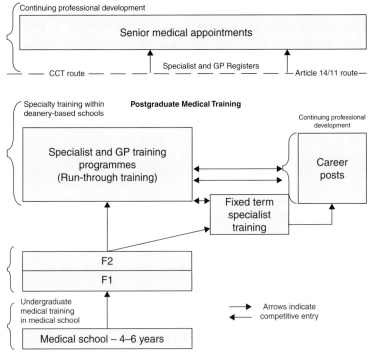

Continuing professional development

Senior medical appointments

CCT route — — — — Specialist and GP Registers — — — Article 14/11 route—

Specialty training within deanery-based schools

Postgraduate Medical Training

Continuing professional development

Specialist and GP training programmes (Run-through training)

Career posts

Fixed term specialist training

F2

F1

Undergraduate medical training in medical school

Arrows indicate competitive entry

Medical school – 4–6 years

Figure 10.1 An outline of postgraduate surgical training (reproduced with permission from Modernising Medical Careers, September 2007). CCT, Certificate of Completion of Training. However, due to its very nature, surgical training is changing all the time so see page 140 for tips on how to stay up to date

2. As a medical student badger your mentors to see if they need help in their audits. Consultants are often too busy to collect data and are more than happy to let you do it. Not only does this give you invaluable experience in clinical governance, but may also get your name on a publication.

3. Read scientific journals and newspapers. Many are now available online. This keeps you up to date with medical news, and often you are able to send in comments and letters to journals, which again leads to publication.

4. Take as many opportunities as you can to give presentations. This not only raises your profile but will also give you experience in talking to large numbers of people.

At a national or international level this scores points when applying for jobs.

5. Consider the advantages and disadvantages of an intercalated BSc degree. This could be an ideal time to demonstrate an interest in surgery by selecting a relevant topic such as anatomy, physiology or pathology.

6. Play an active role in student life during your time in medical school, by joining surgical societies and other student groups and bodies. This can provide managerial and team-working skills that will significantly enhance your CV.

7. Organize an elective in your chosen surgical field. This will offer you an invaluable insight into your future career.

8. Seek and apply for as many prizes, awards and scholarships as you can find. There are many more than you think out there and often these are given out by groups external to your medical school.

9. Take every opportunity there is to teach others or to get involved with projects that involve teaching.

10. Keep a logbook of all your practical procedures, theatre sessions, clinics attended, interesting patients and reflect upon these experiences. It might seem like a bind, but assessors take this very seriously and so should you. Pay particular attention to manual dexterity skills – it is not easy to start with. Some 99% of students have the necessary hand–eye coordination, but some find that they simply cannot form knots, even after much practice. Surgery may not be the best career choice in these circumstances!

KEEPING UP TO DATE

At a time when things are changing rapidly, the best advice we can give you is to stay up to date. The internet is your lifeline to enable you to do this. Here are the top ten websites you need to familiarize yourself with:

1. General Medical Council (www.gmc-uk.org)
2. Medical Training Application Service (www.mtas.nhs.uk)

3. Modernising Medical Careers (www.mmc.nhs.uk)
4. British Medical Association (www.bma.org.uk)
5. Association of Surgeons of Great Britain and Ireland (www.asgbi.org.uk)
6. Association of Surgeons in Training (www.asit.org)
7. Royal College of Surgeons of England (www.rcseng.ac.uk)
8. The Intercollegiate Surgical Curriculum Project (www.iscp.ac.uk)
9. Postgraduate Medical Education and Training Board (www.pmetb.org.uk)
10. Intercollegiate Committee for Basic Surgical Training (www.icbst.org).

Summary

- Take control of your own learning.
- Be around, and get involved with the team.
- Re-read and memorize those top tips!
- When things change rapidly around you, stay up to date.

INDEX

ABCDE approach   34, 35–6
absorbable sutures   68, 69, 70
AC *see* alternating current
access to operating theatres   38
active electrodes   93–4, 119
adhesives   74, 75
airborne pathogens   41
air flow   41
air pressure   41
airway
   ABCDE approach   35
   maintenance   30–2
   preoperative assessment   8–9
alcohol-based preparations   119
alcohol consumption   7
alimentary system   5
alkylphenols   23
allergies   5
alternating current (AC)   88, 89
American Society of Anesthesiologists
      (ASA) physical status
      classification system   3
amine ester   23
aminosteroids   23
anaesthesia   20–37
   desirable drug properties   21
   drugs   21–5
   general   20, 25–6, 33–6
   induction and maintenance   33–6
   inhalational drugs   22
   intravenous drugs   22–5
   observation   47–8
   previous history   6
   procedures and equipment   29–32
   regional   20, 26–9

risk and past medical history   3
   routes of administration   21
   stages   20–1
   techniques   25–9
anaesthetic machine   32
anaesthetic room layout   36–7
anaesthetists   44
analgesics   13, 23
antacids   14
antibiotics   6, 14, 74
anticholinergics   14, 24–5
anticholinesterase   23
antiemetics   14
antimuscarinics   23, 25
antiseptic agents   52–3
anxiolytics   13
argon plasma gas coagulation   108
artery forceps   62, 63
arthritis   113
arthroscopy   113
arylcyclohexylamines   23
ASA *see* American Society of
      Anesthesiologists
aseptic zones   40
aspirin   12
assessments (preoperative)   1–11
assisting the surgeon   84–5
Association of Surgeons of Great
      Britain and Ireland   141
Association of Surgeons in Training   141
atoms   87
attendance   125–6
audits   139
auxiliaries   45
awards   140

Babcock intestinal forceps   62
bags   116
benzodiazepines   23
benzylisoquinolinium   23
Betadine   53
Bier's block   26
biopolar electrosurgery   95–6
blades   117
blended mode   90, 98–9
blood vessel coagulation   98
blunt needles   71
bone   94, 101
bowel preparation   12
braided sutures   69, 70
breathing
    ABCDE approach   35
    airway maintenance   30–2
    preoperative airway assessment
        8–9
British Medical Association   141
brush cleaning   52, 53–4
bupivocaine   23
butterfly sutures   75

capacitive coupling   118
carbonaceous deposits   93–4
carbon dioxide lasers   110
carbon dioxide in pneumoperitoneum
        creation   103–4, 107
carboxy-haemoglobin   120
cardiovascular system medical history
        3–4
careers in surgery   138–40
C-arm image intensifier   121, 122
catgut   69
catheters   17
Cavitron Ultrasonic Surgical Aspirator
        (CUSA)   111
CCT *see* Certificate of Completion of
        Training
central nerve blocks   27–8
Certificate of Completion of Training
        (CCT)   139
changing rooms   137
checks (pre-anaesthetic)   33–4
chlorhexidine gluconate   53
cholecystectomy   102, 107
circuits   88

circulating staff   45
circulation in ABCDE approach   35
clean zones   40, 116
clerking patients   131, 135
clinical waste bags   116
clinic top tips   136
closing surgical gowns   59–60
Clostridium difficile   123
coagulation   97, 98
collagen   73
colonic resection   103
colour codes for hats   43, 47, 137
complications (postoperative)   18
conductive objects   119
confidentiality   129, 135
consent   10–11, 12
contact lenses   120
contact monitoring   118
contaminated waste bags   116
counts of equipment   62, 65, 117
critical care areas   15–16
current   88, 89, 90
curved scissors   63
CUSA *see* Cavitron Ultrasonic Surgical
        Aspirator
cut-down technique   103
cutting in electrosurgery   97–8
cutting needles   71
cyanoacrylate   74
cystoscopy   108

daily rounds   128
daily routine   127–9
day case surgery   17
day of surgery   12–13
Deaver retractor   64
DEEP PIT OF mnemonic   132
dehydration   49
delicate cases in bipolar electrosurgery
        96
dental work   8
depolarizing muscle relaxants   23, 24
desiccation   97, 99
design of operating theatres   41–3
diabetic patients   4, 12
diathermy *see* electrosurgery
diathermy wands   64, 93
dipolar sensing electrosurgery   108

direct current (DC)   88
dirty linen bags   116
dirty zones   116
disability in ABCDE approach   36
discharge
    critical care area   15–16
    postoperative care   17
disposal zones   40
dissecting forceps   63
dissecting scissors   62
donning scrubs   46
donning surgical gowns   56–7
drains   17
drapes   65
dress code   134
drugs
    anaesthetic   21–5
    history   5–6
    preoperative   13–14
    recreational   8

ear, nose and throat (ENT)   111
elasticity of sutures   68
elective procedures   1–2
electrical burns   118
electrical principles   87–90
electrocautery   91
electrodes   93–5, 118, 119
electromagnetic spectrum   89, 90
electron flow   87–8
electronic note systems   128
electrons   110
electrosurgery   86–101
    active electrodes   93–4
    advantages   86
    biopolar electrosurgery   95–6
    blended mode   98–9
    coagulation (fulguration)   97, 98
    cutting   97–8
    desiccation   97, 99
    electrical principles   87–90
    electrocautery   91
    fulguration   97, 98
    hazards   118–19
    laparoscopy   107–8
    monopolar electrosurgery   92–5
    practical tips   99–101
    return electrodes   94–5

surgical smoke hazards   120
    therapeutic effects   96–9
emergency procedures   1–2
endocrine system medical history   4
endogenous agonists   24
endoscopes   108–9
endosurgery   108–9
endotracheal intubation   8–9, 31–2
ENT   111
Entonox   23
epidural anaesthesia   27–8
equipment
    anaesthesia   29–32
    surgical instruments   61–71
eschar   93–4, 101, 119
ethers   23
etiquette   45–9, 137
examinations (preoperative
    assessments)   8–9
exhaustion   134
exogenous agonists   24
exposure in ABCDE approach   36
extracurricular activities   129
eye protection   120

fainting   48–9
family history   6–7
fatty tissues   94, 101
femoral nailing   121
fibroblasts   73
fingernails   12, 51, 52
fire   120
firm, your role in the   130–2
flammable materials   119
follow-up (postoperative period)   17–18
footwear   46, 116, 137
forceps   62–3, 94
formal teaching programme   128
foundation programme   137–8
foundation year   1 doctors   131, 136
frequencies of electrosurgical
    generators   89–90
fulguration (coagulation)   97, 98

gases
    anaesthetic inhalation drugs   22
    laparoscopy   103–4, 107
    toxic gases   120

general anaesthesia   20, 25–6, 33–6
General Medical Council   140
generator settings for electrosurgery
      96–9
genitourinary system medical history   5
getting to know everyone   126, 127, 131
gloves and gloving   57–9, 116
glove sizes   59
glue   74, 75
gowns
      closing   59–60
      donning   56–7
      lead   121, 122

haematological system medical
      history   5
haemostasis   73
hair removal   13
halogenated hydrocarbons   23
handling ability of sutures   68
handovers   131
hand towel technique   55–6
hand-washing   52–5
Harmonic Scalpel   111, 112
hats   43, 47, 116, 137
HDU see high-dependency units
healing stages for wounds   72–3
health   115–23
Health and Safely at Work Act, 1974
      115
HEPA see high-efficiency particulate air
heparin   11
hereditary conditions   6–7
high-dependency units (HDU)   16
high-efficiency particulate air (HEPA)
      filters   41
high-frequency current   90
history   2–8
hobbies   129
hypercarbia   107

identification badges (ID badges)   43,
      46, 47
image interpretation skills   128
imidazoles   23
induction   14, 33–6
infectious diseases   122–3
inflammation   73

inhalational anaesthetics   22, 23
INR see international normalized ratio
instruments   61–71
instrument ties   76–9
insulated forceps   94
insulation failure   118
insulin   12
insulin-dependent diabetic patients   12
intensive therapy units (ITU)   16
intensivist   17
intercalated BSc degrees   140
Intercollegiate Committee for Basic
      Surgical Training   141
The Intercollegiate Surgical Curriculum
      Project   141
intermittently pulsed high-frequency
      current   90
international normalized ratio (INR)   11
Internet   140–1
interventional endoscopy   109
intestinal forceps   62
intramuscular anaesthetics   25
intraoperative period health and safety
      issues   119
intraperitoneal pressure   103–4, 107
intravenous (IV) anaesthetics   22–5
intravenous regional anaesthesia
      (IVRA)   26–7
investigations (preoperative
      assessments)   9–10
ionizing radiation   121–2
Ionizing Radiation (Medical Exposure)
      Regulations (IRMER), 2000   121
ITU see intensive therapy units
IV see intravenous
IVRA see intravenous regional
      anaesthesia

jewellery   12, 51
joints   113
journal clubs   135–6
journals   139

ketamine   23
keyhole surgery see minimal access
      surgery
kidney dishes   65, 117
knee joint   113

knots
    number to tie   84
    practicing   76-9
    security   68
    surgical   80-4
KTP lasers   110

laminar flow systems   41-2
Langenbeck retractor   64
laparoscopy   102-8
laryngeal mask airway (LMA)   30-1
laryngoscope   30, 31
laser surgery   109-11, 120-1
layout of operating theatres   38-40
lead gowns   121, 122
lidocaine   23
LMA *see* laryngeal mask airway
local anaesthetics   29
location of operating theatres   38
logbooks   140

MAC *see* minimum alveolar
    concentration
McIndoe non-toothed forceps   62
macrophages   73
maintenance of general anaesthesia
    33-6
malignant obstructions   109
Mallampati classification   9
Management of Health and Safety at
    Work Regulations, 1999   115
manipulation under anaesthesia (MUA)
    121
manual dexterity   140
marking of operation site   13
masks   51, 116
maturation stage of wound healing   73
Mayo dissecting scissors   62
medical confidentiality   129, 135
Medical Training Application Service
    (MTAS)   138, 140
medications *see* drugs
memory of sutures   68
meniscal tears   113
met-haemoglobin   120
methicillin-resistant *Staphylococcus
    aureus* (MRSA)   123
methyl methacrylate   120

MEWS *see* modified early warning
    score
minimal access surgery   102-14
    arthroscopy   113
    endosurgery   108-9
    laparoscopy   102-8
    laser surgery   109-11, 120-1
    ultrasonic dissection   111-13
minimum alveolar concentration (MAC)
    number   22
MMC *see* Modernising Medical Careers
mnemonics   132-3
Modernising Medical Careers (MMC)
    137, 141
modified early warning score (MEWS)
    chart   16
monitoring of general anaesthesia   35-6
monoamine oxidase inhibitors   6
monofilaments sutures   69, 70
monopolar electrosurgery   92-5
Morris retractor   64
MRSA (methicillin-resistant
    Staphylococcus aureus)   123
MTAS *see* Medical Training Application
    Service
MUA *see* manipulation under
    anaesthesia
multidisciplinary meetings   129
muscle in electrosurgery   94, 100, 101
muscle relaxants   23, 24
musculoskeletal system medical
    history   5
myocardial infarction   4
myofibroblasts   73

nail varnish   12
narcotics (opioids)   22, 23, 24
National Confidential Enquiry into
    Patient Outcome and Death
    (NCEPOD) scoring   2
National Institute for Health and
    Clinical Excellence (NICE)   9-10
natural material sutures   69
natural orifice transluminal endoscopic
    surgery (NOTES)   109
NCEPOD *see* National Confidential
    Enquiry into Patient Outcome
    and Death

needle holders   66
needles   71, 117
needlestick injuries   117–18
neurological system medical history   4
neutrophils   73
newspapers   139
NICE *see* National Institute for Health
    and Clinical Excellence
nitrous oxide   23
non-absorbable sutures   68, 69, 70
non-depolarizing muscle relaxants
    23, 24
non-steroidal anti-inflammatory drugs
    (NSAIDS)   12, 23
nonswaged needles   71
non-toothed forceps   62, 63
NOTES *see* natural orifice transluminal
    endoscopic surgery
note taking   128, 131
NSAIDS *see* non-steroidal anti-
    inflammatory drugs
nurses   44
nutrition   5

obesity   5
ODPs *see* operating department
    practitioners
on-calls   133
oncology   111
one-handed reef knots   80–3
operating department practitioners
    (ODPs)   44–5
operating theatres   38–49
    aseptic zones   40
    clean zones   40
    design   41–3
    disposal zones   40
    etiquette   45–9, 137
    layout   38–40
    patient preparation   11–14
    protective zones   39
    staff   43–5
    sterile (aseptic zones)   40
    temperature   41
    top tips   136–7
operation notes   85
opioid receptors   24
opioids   22, 23, 24

optical fibre cables   103
oral contraceptives   5–6
orthopaedic surgery   41–2, 121
outreach nurses   17
overnight stay surgery   17

pacemakers   94–5
paracetamol   23
past medical history   3–5
PDS *see* polydioxanone sutures
perioperative care   1–19
    anaesthesia induction   14
    electrosurgery safety measures
        118–19
    intraoperative period   14
    postoperative period   14–18
    preoperative assessments   1–11
    referrals   1–2
    theatre preparation   11–14
peripheral blocks   29
peri-prosthetic infections   41
Perma-hand sutures   70
physiology   133
physiotherapists   17
plastic surgery   111
plate burns   118
pneumoperitoneum   103, 107
polydioxanone sutures (PDS)   70
polyfilament sutures   69, 70
Polyglactin   910 (Vicryl) sutures   70
polypropylene (Prolene) sutures   70
porters   45
ports for laparoscopy   104–5
Postgraduate Medical Education and
    Training Board   141
postgraduate surgical training outline
    139
postoperative period   14–18
    care   16–17
    complications   6, 18
    critical care areas   15–16
    electrosurgery safety measures   119
    follow up   17–18
    recovery period   15
    rounds   129
povidone iodine   53
power   88, 89
pre-anaesthetic checks   33–4

preoperative assessments 1–11
  consent 10–11
  examination 8–9
  history 2–8
  investigations 9–10
  ward rounds 46
preoperative electrosurgery safety
    measures 118–19
preoperative medications 13–14
pre-registration house officers (PRHO)
  137
presentations 139–40
PRHO *see* pre-registration house
  officers
primary beam 122
prizes 140
procedure-specific wrist bands 13
Prolene sutures 70
proliferation stage of wound healing
  73
protective zones 39
publications 139
punctuality 134
pure high-frequency current 90

questions 49, 84–5, 130, 133
quivers 65

radiation safety 121–2
radiofrequencies 89, 90
radio-opaque strips 65, 117
rapid sequence induction (RSI) 32
recovery period 15
recreational drug use 8
reef knots 80–3
referrals for surgical procedures 1–2
refreshments 136
regional anaesthesia 20, 26–9
resistance 88, 89
respiratory system medical history 4
respiratory tract infections 4, 12
retractors 64
return electrodes 92, 94–5, 118, 119
reversal agents 23, 24–5
reverse cutting needles 71
risk assessments 115
round-bodied needles 71
rounds *see* ward rounds

routes of administration for anaesthetic
    drugs 21
Royal College of Surgeons of England
  141
RSI *see* rapid sequence induction

safety 115–23
scalpels 64–5, 111, 112
scholarships 140
scientific journals 139
scissors 62, 63
scratch pads 94, 101
screening time of radiation exposure
  121
scrubbing up 48, 51–60, 137
  closing surgical gowns 59–60
  donning surgical gowns 56–7
  gloving 57–9
  hand towel technique 55–6
  hand-washing 52–5
scrub nurses 44
scrubs 46, 116, 137
secondary intention 73, 74
senior house officers (SHO) 137
seniors (top tips) 135
sharps 117–18
shaving 13
SHO *see* senior house officers
shoes 46, 116, 137
silk (Perma-hand) sutures 70
skin
  adhesives 74, 75
  brushing 53
  laser surgery hazards 120
  lesions 98
sliding scale 12
smoke hazards 120
smoking history 7
social history 7–8
specialty training (ST) 138
Spencer-Well artery forceps 62, 63
spider haemangiomas 99
spinal anaesthesia 27–8
spongeholders 63
ST *see* specialty training
staff in theatre 43–5
Staphylococcus aureus 123
staples 75

step down units   16
sterile drapes   65
sterile zones   40
sterilization by laparoscopy   105
Steristrips   75
steroids   6
STOP moment   13, 117
straight scissors   63
student life   140
subcutaneous anaesthetics   25
sucker tubes   120
surgeons   43–4, 115–23
surgical gowns
    closing   59–60
    donning   56–7
    lead   121, 122
surgical history   6
surgical instruments   61–71
surgical knot tying   80–4
surgical masks   116
surgical smoke hazards   120
suture needles   71
suture scissors   62
sutures
    butterfly   75
    classification   67–71
    ideal   66–7
    material properties   67, 68
    sizing   67, 68
suturing
    art of   72–85
    practicing   76–9
    techniques   76–80
    tips   79–80
swabs   62, 65, 117
swaged needles   71
sympathomimetic amine   23
synthetic sutures   69

talking   116
teachers   125–6
teeth   8
telangiectasias   99
temperature of operating theatre   41
tensile strength of sutures   68
tetanus immunization   74
theatre managers   44
theatre nurses   44

theatre practitioners   44
theatres *see* operating theatres
The Intercollegiate Surgical Curriculum
    Project   141
therapeutic electrosurgical effects
    96–9
thermoluminescent dosimeter (TLD)
    badges   122
thyroid shields   121
thyromental distance   9
tissue forceps   63
tissue reactivity to sutures   68
TLD *see* thermoluminescent dosimeter
toothed forceps   62, 63
top tips   133–7
tourniquets   26–7
towel clips   65
toxic gases   120
trainees   45
transfer locations   16
traumatic injuries   113
Trendelenburg position   103
triad of anaesthesia   25
trocar   104
typical day   127–9

ultrasonic dissection   111–13
unidirectional air flow   41
urinary catheters   17
urology   111

valuables   39, 47
VATS *see* video-assisted thoracoscopic
    surgery
ventilation of theatres   41, 116
Veress needles   103, 104
vessel coagulation   98
Vicryl sutures   70
video-assisted thoracoscopic surgery
    (VATS)   108
VITAMIN D mnemonic   132–3
volatile liquid hazards   120
voltage   88, 89

ward rounds
    daily   128
    note taking   136
    postoperative period   129

presenting patients   131, 135
turning up to   130
ward sisters   135
ward top tips   135–6
warfarin   6, 11
waste bags   61–2
wavelengths
electromagnetic spectrum   90
lasers   110
websites   140–1

wound drains   17
wounds
assessment and management   73–6
closure methods   74–6
healing stages   72–3
wrist bands   13

X-rays   121–2

YAG lasers   110